Beautiful Hands & Nails Naturally

Fran Manos

Avery Publishing Group
Garden City Park, New York

Text Illustrator: John Wincek
Front Cover Photograph: PhotoDisc
Cover Design: William Gonzalez
Typesetting: Elaine V. McCaw
In-House Editor: Joanne Abrams

Avery Publishing Group
120 Old Broadway
Garden City Park, NY 11040
1-800-548-5757

Publisher's Cataloging-in-Publication

Manos, Fran.
    Beautiful hands and nails, naturally : achieving and
maintaining youthful, radiantly healthy hands and nails/
Fran Manos.
    p. cm.
    Includes bibliographical references and index.
    ISBN: 0-89529-838-4

    1. Nails (Anatomy)—Care and hygiene. 2. Hand—Care and
hygiene. 3. Beauty, Personal. 4. Manicuring. I. Title.

RL94.M36 1998   646.727
                                                 QBI97-41616

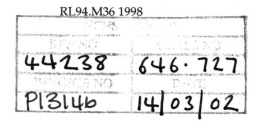
Printed in the United States of America

10 9 8 7 6 5 4 3 2 1

Beautiful
Hands&Nails
Naturally

Contents

To Jim, my husband, for his love and good-humored support of my nail obsession. To my mom, Gwyneth Lyon, for her belief in me. And in memory of my father, William Lyon.

Preface

I'm going to assume that you've picked up this book because you're not satisfied with your hands and nails—both with their appearance and with what they say about you. You may have tried for years, on and off, to have consistently well-groomed hands and nails only to find that the polish always seems to chip, that the nails tear or break, and that the cuticles get ragged. Perhaps you are also plagued by spots that appear on the backs of your hands. (Sometimes I think it's the spots that are the final straw!) It's so maddening—especially if you've painstakingly followed the standard manicure advice offered in so many books and magazine articles. You may even have a shoebox packed with all the bottles of polish that you've tried and found wanting. Because, let's face it, even the prettiest polish isn't pretty on a set of chipped nails graced with a ragged hangnail or two. And if you have rough, grimy calluses and nails dotted with white flecks—and perhaps some nail ridging as well—you may wish you could hide your hands in brown paper bags.

I know that nail care can be so frustrating that you may be tempted to hide your nail problems under artificial nails. But you'll soon see why antifungal medications are usually sold next to artificial nail products. And then you'll realize why the artificial nail route may not be the path that you want to take!

At this point, you're probably ready for a new approach to hand and nail care. This is where *Beautiful Hands and Nails, Naturally* comes in. It was when I learned to care for my own fragile nails that I devised an effective alternative to polish-based nail care. This program not only works, but leaves your nails in better condition—not worse—than they were in when you started.

Beautiful Hands and Nails, Naturally begins by looking at the basic anatomy of hands and nails, as well as the delicate structure of the skin itself. Armed with this knowledge, you'll understand why certain common hand- and nail-care practices are unwise, and why other procedures really work.

In Chapter 2, you'll plunge right into the basics of the Beautiful Hands and Nails Regimen, a simple daily four-step program. I think you'll find it fun, and I know that the sooner you can see your nails becoming prettier and your hands becoming smoother, the better!

In Chapter 3, you'll discover one of the secrets to beautiful, healthy nails: healthy cuticles. Specific manicure techniques as well as gentle cuticle smoothers will shape up your cuticles in no time.

Chapter 4 presents everything you need to know to have perfectly filed nails. Even if you're "all thumbs" when it comes to filing, step-by-step instructions will guide you in creating beautifully shaped nails, and in keeping them that way. In this chapter, you'll also learn to make Beeswax Nail Spackle, my secret weapon in the war against chips and splits.

While nice, neat, "invisible" nails and smooth cuticles are nothing to sneeze at, in Chapter 5, you'll learn how to give your nails zip and pizzazz. You'll clean and whiten them, shine them, and color them—all naturally. You'll also learn how to harden your nails using fragrant natural resins, not formaldehyde!

No, I haven't forgotten about hands, as you'll see in Chapter 6. Here, you'll find simple ways to both protect and heal your hard-working hands. If your hands are weather-beaten and perhaps sun-damaged, I think you'll enjoy these treatments for smoothing and softening that delicate skin. These are treatments that not only make your hands look good, but also feel good as you use them.

Finally, in Chapter 7, you'll learn how to care for your hands and nails from the inside out. Plenty of exercise, a nutritious diet, and a good night's sleep can make a big difference in health and appearance. And, of course, a healthy lifestyle will improve your general feeling of well-being—a sure way to look great.

As you begin using the Beautiful Hands and Nails Regimen, as well as enjoying my specific treatments and therapies, you'll be delighted to discover that this program produces *consistent results*. Never again will you have nicely polished nails on Saturday night right after your manicure, only to have a disaster literally on your hands by Monday, after the polish has chipped.

Follow my easy four-part regimen, and you will have beautiful hands and nails, naturally. I'll think you'll really be pleased.

Beautiful Hands and Nails, Naturally

Introduction

Smooth, soft hands and perfectly groomed nails. Haven't you always wished they were yours? Nails with the translucent sheen of the inside of a seashell, or as pretty as flower petals. I know I used to dream about them, and perhaps you have, too. Hands and nails the French would call *soigné*, or perfectly, meticulously groomed. The last refined detail in your overall appearance.

I used to dream about such hands, because, for years, my nails were always first prize winners in the Worst Nails in the World contest. To put it mildly, they were problem nails. It wasn't just a matter of an occasional split or chip. Sometimes the whole tip of a nail would tear off like paper. And then there were the hangnails, the dry and hard cuticles, and, of course, the calluses. Grimy calluses were a persistent problem for me. Smears of ink, pencil dust, photocopier toner, carbon copy smudges—you name it—were ground into my fingertips after a day's work. These unsightly stains resisted washing with mere soap. I found that even the papers I handled every day wicked moisture from my fingertips, leaving them cracked and roughened as though I made my living loading bales of hay, instead of working in a modern office.

Nail polish, especially, presented problems for me. I always seemed to be in the process of shakily applying the polish, fanning my hands as I waited for it to dry, smudging it, and then, of course, touching up the chips. Occasionally, a big glob of polish would land on a finger, missing the nail entirely.

But I struggled along, carefully following the usual manicure routine of applying polish and removing it and trying to shore up my nails with nail hardeners. I kept trying because I had been thoroughly indoctrinated by articles in women's magazines, and, to be honest, by my friends. Beauty experts and peers alike had convinced me that *real* women have talons—long, curling-over, Dragon Lady claws, sometimes encrusted with rhinestones. Claws that could draw blood if they had to.

Sometimes I gave up entirely, in disgust, and abandoned my hands and nails to fate and the elements. I won't divulge all the gory details, but my nails quickly became a rogue's gallery of broken nails, hangnails, short nails, long nails—horrible nails.

Somewhere along the line, I developed a nail-biting habit. In retrospect, there was nothing surprising in this, as any roughness on cuticles and nails tends to act as a natural focal point for nervous behavior. But it still was discouraging.

Just when I thought that my hands and nails couldn't possibly get any worse, I noticed the beginning of so-called "age spots" on the backs of my hands. Feeling my hair stand on end, I realized that my hands were beginning to resemble my mother's hands. But she was seventy-two and I, well, I have a long way to go before I'm seventy-two!

I finally started to realize that traditional nail-care advice simply didn't work for me. The light finally dawned. It didn't matter what the experts said—my fragile nails were wrecked by the trauma of the repeated application and removal of nail polish. The harsh solvents in nail polish remover, especially, left my nails dried out and waiting to split. And nail hardeners, rather than making my nails stronger, actually seemed to make them *brittle*. Could this be possible? Just as frustrating, I could diligently push back my cuticles all day long, but they remained dry and ragged.

I also realized that my personal ideal of feminine beauty differed from that portrayed in fashion magazines. I looked at the graceful hands of women in Renaissance paintings, and thought how truly lovely they were. I tried to imagine Mona Lisa with long red nails, and somehow the effect was not the same. I thought of the goddesses and cherubs portrayed by the painter Titian. They seemed to glow with a pearly, inner radiance. Their beauty arose from the enhanced natural beauty of their skin and hair, not from any blatantly artificial color.

When I picked up a bottle of the nail hardener I was using and read the list of ingredients, I was startled to see chemicals that would be right at home in a toxic waste dump. At that point, something really clicked. I was tired of letting the unkempt, roughened appearance of my hands and nails detract from my appearance. There had to be a better way. Fragile nails and problem hands needed special care. I decided to learn how to have pretty nails without using polishes and nail hardeners. I decided to use Mona Lisa—not Cher—as my inspiration. I wanted to see if going "natural" would work for me.

I began my quest by studying every bit of information I could find on hand and nail care. Herbal treatments, aromatherapy, raw juice therapy, recipes from the ladies of the court of Louis XIV—you name it, I tried it. I began to experiment with homemade creams, lotions, and potions. I took vitamins. I tried everything from paraffin treatments and mashed bananas to grapefruit peels tied to the backs of my hands. (Fortunately, my husband is used to my peculiarities, and said nothing.) I investigated and questioned every home remedy I could find concerning nails—and there are a lot of them! (In the coming chapters, I think you'll be interested to see some popular wives' tales—supposedly tried-and-true remedies—debunked.) Nutrition quickly zoomed to the top of my list as a subject worthy of study when I began to realize the crucial part it played in the growth of strong, healthy nails.

My aim was to devise a method of natural hand and nail care that would be simple, effective, and practical for real women living busy lives. This took time because, as I've mentioned, I had been brainwashed to believe that polish-based nail care was the only way to go.

At first, I worried about my new natural approach to hand and nail care. If I didn't use a nail hardener, wouldn't my nails fall apart? Might they even fall off? Didn't fragile, baby-soft nails like mine *require* a hardener, a bottom coat, a middle coat, and a top coat? A glance at my nails, however, told me that they couldn't get much worse than they already were, and that I should follow my instincts—that natural was best. So I chucked the hardener, the bottom coat, and the top coat, and redoubled my efforts to learn what was really effective in hand and nail care.

The result of these efforts is the four-part regimen of natural care for hands and nails that you will find in this book. My main criterion for any hand and nail care treatment has been: does it work and, most important, does it work in *real life*? I don't have the time or money for trips to health spas, or for regular appointments at a manicurist. That may be true for you, too. On the other hand, I don't mind spending *some* time on my hands and nails, as long my efforts yield results. I have also had to consider just how "natural" I want my regimen to be. The word "natural" has been so distorted by advertisers that it's difficult to know what it means anymore. In this book, it means not using nail polish, nail polish remover, chemical nail hardeners or cuticle removers, or, of course, artificial nails. Beyond this, I feel that the use of some commercial products is not only acceptable, but is advisable, as in the case with sunscreens.

Are these treatments truly effective? I'm somewhat skeptical by nature, and as a modern woman, I feel that I've seen everything—twice. When I began to care for my nails naturally, I didn't know what to expect. But I have found that these treatments do work—to a degree that still surprises and delights me. You will see a noticeable difference in your nails' appearance after just a few days of the Beautiful Hands and Nails Regimen. After one month, your nails will be significantly improved, even transformed. Remember, though, that the realistic timetable for improvement depends on the initial condition of your nails, on your nails' intrinsic softness or hardness, and on your own diligence in following the program. It takes about six months to grow an entirely new nail, depending on your metabolism, the quality of your diet, and the season of the year. All the more reason to start right away!

If you are a refugee from the land of artificial nails—welcome. As you can imagine, as a fan of natural nails, I feel that gluing on artificial nails is one of the worst things you can do to your hands. So before starting on this regimen, I recommend that you have your nails examined by a dermatologist. Fungal infections can develop in real nails trapped under artificial ones, and sometimes the top layer of the nails can be weakened when the artificial nail is peeled off. So make sure you have nothing seriously amiss before embarking on a course of natural hand and nail care.

While these treatments are aimed at those who wish to have naturally pretty nails, I don't at all mean to offend those readers who enjoy using polish. It's a valid fashion look—it's just not for everybody. If you do wear nail polish, I urge you to give your nails a breather now and then and lavish on them some of the treatments found in this book. And if your hands are beginning to look a little too much like your mother's for comfort, in the coming pages you will find a treasure trove of effective turn-back-the-clock treatments designed to restore smoothness, softness, and even tone.

So if you desire pretty hands and smooth, translucent nails—*without* using divinylbenzene copolymer carbomer 941 or benzophenone-1—read on! Your hands and nails really can be beautiful, naturally.

Troubleshooting for Hand and Nail Problems

*A*s you will learn in the following chapters, a simple four-part program will allow you to maintain the health and beauty of your hands and nails and to avoid a number of problems. However, should you have specific problems right now, the table below will help you pinpoint possible causes, as well as suggest a variety of strategies and treatments that can help bring relief and also act as preventives for the future. Once you have identified the desired strategy, turn to the appropriate chapter as necessary to learn how you can make it a part of your hand- and nail-care regimen.

At-a-Glance Therapy for Common Hand and Nail Problems

Problems	Possible Causes	Helpful Treatments and Strategies
Age Spots	• Long-term sun exposure.	• Use the natural treatments presented in Chapter 6 to fade age spots. Also try the exfoliants discussed in that chapter, as they will smooth the rough, spotted skin, making the spots appear less pronounced.

Problems	Possible Causes	Helpful Treatments and Strategies
Age Spots (continued)		• During the day, protect your hands from the harmful effects of the sun by using a moisturizer that contains a sunscreen. When spending considerable time out of doors—especially during late morning and early afternoon— use a regular sunscreen to provide added protection.
Brittle Nails	• Poor diet—especially one inadequate in essential fatty acids; vitamins, including biotin; and/or sulfur. • Long-term sun exposure. • Use of commercial nail hardeners.	• Make sure your diet contains foods that provide all the nutrients necessary for nail health. (See Chapter 7.) • Protect your nails from the effects of the sun by always wearing your nail protector. (See Chapter 2.) • When moisturizing your hands, be sure to also moisturize the nails. (See Chapter 2.) • Avoid the use of nail hardeners, many of which contain formaldehyde, a product that actually dehydrates the nails.
Cracked Fingertips	• Exposure to drying soaps, detergents, or chemicals. • Insufficient use of moisturizers.	• Protect your hands with rubber gloves when doing household chores. • Use your moisturizer in the morning and often throughout the day. It is especially important to moisturize after every exposure to hot water. The fingertips contain very few sebaceous glands— the glands that produce an oil which "waterproofs" skin. Therefore, they require extra protection. • Rub small amounts of petroleum jelly or lip balm into your fingertips throughout the day.

Problems	Possible Causes	Helpful Treatments and Strategies
Cracked Fingertips (continued)		• When performing office chores that involve touching paper, moisturize your hands frequently, and consider using rubber finger guards when sorting and filing. Paper wicks moisture from the skin, leaving it dry and uncomfortable.
Discolored, Yellowed Nails	• Use of nail polish or commercial nail hardeners. • Injury to the nail, such as a blow. • Use of certain medications. • Fungal infection. • Poor circulation. • Smoking. • Aging and long-term exposure to sun.	• Avoid the use of nail polish, as well as the use of other commercial nail products. • Allow any discoloration or other mark caused by trauma to grow out on its own. • Discuss any effects of medication with your doctor. • When fungal infections cause the nail to be cloudy or white, see your doctor immediately, as a medication will probably be needed to clear the infection. (See Chapter 7.) • Get regular exercise to improve your circulation. This will give you pink nail beds and healthier-looking nails. (See Chapter 7.) • Quit smoking (and not just for the health of your nails!). Smoking decreases circulation to the fingertips, resulting in pallid nail beds and unhealthy nails. (See Chapter 7.) • Try using a mild hydrogen peroxide bleaching procedure for cleaner, whiter-looking nails. (See Chapter 5.) • Protect your nails from the effects of the sun by always wearing your nail protector. (See Chapter 2.)

Problems	Possible Causes	Helpful Treatments and Strategies
Dry, Rough Skin	• Exposure to drying soaps, detergents, or chemicals. • Insufficient use of moisturizers. • Exposure to hot sun, cold weather, or the drying effects of central heating.	• Protect your hands with rubber gloves when doing household chores. • Use your moisturizer in the morning and often throughout the day. It is especially important to moisturize after every exposure to hot water. This is a vital part of your Beautiful Hands and Nails Regimen. (See Chapter 2.) • The moment the weather turns cold, wear your gloves every time you go outside. • For immediate relief from dry, cracked skin, use the Warm Paraffin Hand Treatment, an effective and soothing softener, and the Intensive Moisturizing Treatment. (See Chapter 6.)
Hangnails	• Simple neglect. • Exposure to drying soaps, detergents, or chemicals. • Picking and biting at cuticle area.	• Follow the Beautiful Hands and Nails Regimen daily. (See Chapter 2.) • Protect your hands with rubber gloves when doing household work. • Massage a dab of Apricot Oil-Lanolin Cuticle Salve into each cuticle every morning and evening. (See Chapter 3.) • Use a cuticle trimmer to prevent the buildup of dry, dead cuticle skin. (See Chapter 3.) • Use effective strategies to kick the nail-biting habit, as these should also help you avoid biting your cuticles. (See Chapter 7.)
Hard, Overgrown Cuticles	• Simple neglect. • Use of commercial nail-care products such as cuticle removers, which can irritate and dry the skin.	• Follow the Beautiful Hands and Nails Regimen daily. (See Chapter 2.) • Massage a dab of Apricot Oil-Lanolin Cuticle Salve into each cuticle every morning and evening. (See Chapter 3.)

Problems	Possible Causes	Helpful Treatments and Strategies
Hard, Overgrown Cuticles (continued)		• Use the Cornmeal Cuticle Smoother twice a week until cuticles become softer and smoother; then use the treatment once a week. (See Chapter 3.) • Use a cuticle trimmer once a week to remove hard, dry skin. (See Chapter 3.)
Inflamed, Infected Skin Around the Nails	• Hangnail infection or overmanipulation of the cuticle. Can be bacterial or fungal in origin. • Overexposure to drying soaps, detergents, or chemicals.	• Try applying undiluted tea tree oil to the affected area. Tea tree oil is a natural antiseptic and will help decrease inflammation. (See Chapter 3.) • If the infection persists, see a dermatologist. An antifungal medication or another medication may be necessary. • Always use gentleness and restraint when pushing back or grooming cuticles. • Protect your hands with rubber gloves when doing household chores.
Itchy, Irritated Skin	• Overexposure to drying soaps, detergents, or chemicals. • Exposure to irritants and potential allergens, such as nickel, latex, rubber, and cosmetic ingredients such as parabens.	• Protect your hands with rubber gloves when doing household chores. • If possible, identify and eliminate the product that is causing the problem. If you don't know the source of the problem, see your dermatologist as soon as possible. (See Chapter 6.)
Nail Ridges	• Heredity. • Poor diet. • Anemia. • Overzealous manicuring.	• Although heredity can't be changed, and some ridging of the nails is normal, buffing with a buffing cream can help smooth ridged nail surfaces. (See Chapter 5.)

Problems	Possible Causes	Helpful Treatments and Strategies
Nail Ridges (continued)		• If nails are heavily ridged, consider using a ridge sander, which can help smooth ridges that run vertically along the nail. These should be used no more than once a month. (See Chapter 4.) • Make sure your diet contains foods that provide all the nutrients necessary for nail health. (See Chapter 7.) • If you have developed ridges for the first time, this may be a sign of anemia. See your doctor. • Use gentleness and restraint when pushing back or grooming cuticles. Vigorous pushing may cause crosswise ridges, bumps, or indentations in the nail surface. (See Chapter 3.)
Slow Nail Growth	• Illness. • Use of certain medications. • Poor diet.	• Once you have recovered from your illness, normal nail growth should resume. • Discuss any effects of medication with your doctor. • Make sure your diet contains foods that provide all the nutrients necessary for nail health. (See Chapter 7.)
Splitting, Peeling Nails	• Heredity. • An allergy to or overuse of nail polish removers. • Poor diet. • Frequent immersion of hands in water. • Exposure to drying soaps, detergents, or chemicals. • Improper nail filing tools or techniques.	• Although heredity can't be changed, you can protect your nails every day with a nail protector, and nourish them every night with a nail nourisher. (See Chapter 2.) • If possible, avoid the use of polish and removers. If you do use nail polish, don't remove it more than once a week, as polish removers strip nails of their natural moisture, leaving

Problems	Possible Causes	Helpful Treatments and Strategies
Splitting, Peeling Nails (continued)		them vulnerable to splitting and peeling. • Make sure your diet contains foods that provide all the nutrients necessary for nail health. (See Chapter 7.) • Protect your hands with rubber gloves when doing household chores. • File your nails gently, using a high-quality nail file—preferably one coated with gem dust. (See Chapter 4.)
Weak, Fragile Nails	• Heredity. • Crash dieting or a poor diet. • Exposure to drying soaps, detergents, or chemicals. • Using nails as "tools" to accomplish tasks. • Long nail length.	• Although heredity can't be changed, you can protect your nails every day with a nail protector, and nourish them every night with a nail nourisher. (See Chapter 2.) This will moisturize your nails, making them more pliable and less likely to break. • Make sure your diet contains foods that provide all the nutrients necessary for nail health. (See Chapter 7). • Protect your hands with rubber gloves when doing chores. • Respect your nails, and avoid using them as scrapers, screwdrivers, or other tools. • Try wearing your nails no longer than fingertip length, and square them off for added stability. If your nails are naturally fragile, long nail lengths may be unrealistic.
White Spots on Nails	• Blows to the nail or excessive pressure to the matrix, the area	• A white spot caused by trauma is nothing to worry about. Allow it to grow out naturally.

Problems	Possible Causes	Helpful Treatments and Strategies
White Spots on Nails (continued)	that generates new nail growth. • Overzealous manicuring with sharp implements.	• Use gentleness and restraint when pushing back or grooming cuticles. Poking under the cuticles with sharp implements can injure the area where new nail cells are emerging, causing spots. (See Chapter 3.)

Chapter 1

Understanding Your Hands and Nails

*B*efore I began studying hand and nail care seriously, like most of us, I took my hands for granted. I never thought about them one way or the other as they folded tortellini for dinner (a hand tour de force if there ever was one), performed the delicate hand ballet involved in knitting lace, or gently stroked the downy fur of a kitten. They were just my hands. They had always been there at the ends of my arms doing what my brain told them to do.

Yet if you think about what your hands do for you, you will see them as the miracle of form and function that they are. For sheer versatility, the human hand has no equal anywhere in the animal kingdom. Think of how stymied you would be if you had paws or hooves. You couldn't use the remote control device to change the channel of your TV, much less build a bookcase, arrange flowers, or play beautiful music on a piano. But as strong and adaptable as hands are, they are also vulnerable to the abuses of time, weather, and everyday life— which is why this book was written. Only by having some knowledge of how your hands—and the nails attached to them—are formed and work can you appreciate their delicacy, and understand how to keep them healthy and beautiful.

This chapter will familiarize you with the basic anatomy of hands, skin, and nails. In the process, you will begin to see how these structures can become damaged, as well as how this damage can often be avoided.

THE HANDS AND SKIN

Someone of a poetic turn might say that the hands are extensions of the soul—a means of reaching out into the world and realizing your dreams. At the very least, the hands are the servants of the brain—physically touching the objects around you, sensing them, and manipulating them. Even the seemingly simple act of holding this book in your hands involves a flurry of detailed communications between hands and brain. For instance—and this was news to me—your hands basically have two grips. Knowing that you want to balance this book in your hands and turn the pages, your brain instructs your hands to use their precision grip, so that the book is handled delicately. Later on, if you pick up a hammer to pound a nail, the brain directs the hand to use its power grip, and the hand becomes an instrument of strength.

What makes your hands—and the skin that covers them— capable of serving you so well? Let's examine each of these structures in turn.

The Anatomy of the Hands

Even a brief glance at the internal structure of hands reveals their mind-boggling complexity. Nerves, muscles, arteries, and veins crisscross one another, looking like a map of the Los Angeles freeway. An elaborate network of tough ligaments and tendons, looking a bit like rubberbands, is poised to respond to the brain's slightest commands. The tendons that connect muscle to bone are encased in lubricated fibrous sheaths that allow the tendons freedom to flex and contract. The ligaments, delicate bands fanning out over and under one another, connect bone to bone. The bones of the hand and wrist—there are twenty-six—are as beautifully shaped as precious jewels, and precisely designed according to their function. For instance, the delicate bones of the fingertips are smoothed and rounded to serve as understructures for the fingernails. (More about nails later in the chapter!)

The Anatomy of the Skin

Covering the hands and protecting them is that organ known as the skin. (Yes, the skin is an organ!) Skin forms a protective barrier between you and the outside world, shielding your internal organs from germs, toxic chemicals, and ultraviolet rays. It is also waterproof, which is fortunate, or taking a bath or shower would be an interesting experience! Skin also regulates body temperature; produces vitamin D for the use of the body; and gathers sensory information from the outside world, thereby enabling the hands to better manipulate the objects to which they come into contact.

Skin is composed of three main layers. (See Figure 1.1.) At the base of the skin is the *subcutaneous layer,* which is made largely of fat cells embedded in loosely bound connective tissue. This layer pads the skin above, helping to absorb blows and pressure. It also serves to insulate the body and keep it warm. The subcutaneous layer differs in thickness according to its location on the body. The layer on the back of the hand is comparatively thin, which is one reason why hands often feel colder than does the rest of the body. And with only a thin supportive fat pad to keep it smooth, the skin on the back of the hand wrinkles easily.

Above the subcutaneous layer is the *dermis,* which contains many of the skin's structures, such as nerves and blood and lymph vessels. This layer also contains the sweat glands, which help to regulate body temperature and excrete wastes; the sebaceous glands, which produce sebum, an oil that waterproofs the skin; and the hair folli-

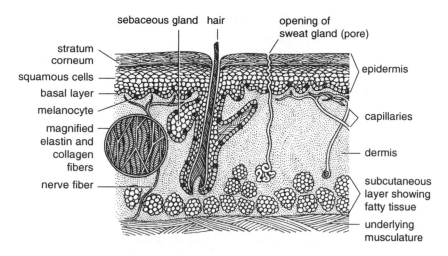

sebaceous gland   hair

opening of
sweat gland (pore)

stratum
corneum

squamous cells

basal layer

melanocyte

magnified
elastin and
collagen
fibers

nerve fiber

epidermis

capillaries

dermis

subcutaneous
layer showing
fatty tissue

underlying
musculature

Figure 1.1 Cross-Section of the Skin

cles. The dermis of the skin on the back of the hand contains few sweat or sebaceous glands compared with the skin on the rest of the body. This is another reason why this area wrinkles and dries so easily.

The dermis contains two vital skin proteins—collagen and elastin. Collagen fibers form a protein net that gives the skin its strength and firmness, while elastin fibers allow the skin to snap back into place after it is stretched. Ultraviolet rays from the sun easily penetrate the dermis, damaging collagen and elastin by causing them to crumble and break. Since most hands are often exposed to the sun, the skin here is particularly vulnerable to sun damage and, yes, wrinkling. That's why later chapters so often mention the importance of shielding your hands with sunscreen.

The bumpy surface of the dermis is rich with capillaries that bring oxygen and nutrients to the next, and outermost, layer of the skin: the *epidermis.* This layer is very thin, and is in a constant state of self-renewal. New skin cells are produced in the lowest level of the epidermis, the *basal layer,* which is in direct contact with the dermis. When the skin cells are produced, they push the cells above them to the surface of the skin, a process that takes about two weeks. As the cells move farther and farther from the life-giving capillaries of the dermis—first to the *squamous layer* (the middle layer of the epidermis), and then to the *stratum corneum* (the outermost layer of the epidermis)—they begin to die, and become drier and flatter. By the time they reach the stratum corneum, or keratin layer, the cells are dead. This layer, which is only about twenty cells thick, sloughs off naturally. In a later chapter, you will learn how this renewal and sloughing process can be speeded up, revealing the fresh skin cells beneath.

There's one more noteworthy feature of the epidermis—noteworthy, that is, for anyone who is interested in having younger-looking skin. The basal layer of the epidermis contains cells called *melanocytes.* These cells produce melanin, the dark-colored pigment of the skin that absorbs the sun's ultraviolet rays, preventing the rays from reaching and damaging the dermis. Years of sun exposure often cause melanin to pool unevenly in the epidermis, resulting in age spots. So here's another good reason to use sunscreen!

THE NAILS

Your fingertips are packed with specialized sensory cells that allow you to experience the world intensely through the sense of touch. The most common of these cells are Meissner's corpuscle, which senses intermittent touch, and Merkel's discs, which sense light, continuous touch. Other corpuscles sense heat, cold, and light and heavy pressure.

This very sensitivity renders the fingertips especially vulnerable to pain. And, of course, the fact that you use your hands to perform an endless variety of tasks—everything from cooking to typing to working in the garden—renders them especially vulnerable to injury. This is why nails are so important. The main function of nails is to protect the fingertips. Let's just imagine—and let's hope it only happens in your imagination—that you smash your thumb with a hammer. Ouch! Without the shield of the thumbnail, the tissue of the thumb could be crushed. This could lead to infection and, ultimately, even to the loss of the finger. While the nail can't protect your thumb from every trauma, it does do an excellent job of shielding it from the damage that can result from everyday wear and tear and from minor accidents.

Nails also help you to pick up and manipulate small objects, and to perform such delicate tasks as threading a needle. Imagine trying to pick up a paperclip, for instance, without fingernails. You would probably feel all thumbs!

The Anatomy of the Nails

The nail itself rests on the *nail bed,* a fleshy area containing a rich network of capillaries that oxygenate and nourish the nail *matrix.* (See Figure 1.2.) This matrix is the area that generates new nail cells. (You'll learn more about nail growth later in this chapter.)

The *lunula* is the white moon-shaped crescent at the base of the nail. This is the visible part of the nail matrix. Often it can be seen only on the thumb. (It is perfectly normal not to see it on the other fingers.) The lunula is white because the matrix is a relatively thick portion of the nail, and therefore blocks out the pink tint of the capillary-rich nail bed.

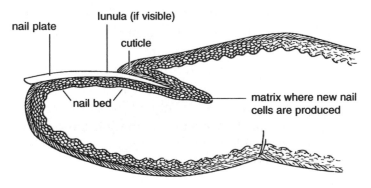

Figure 1.2 Cross-Section of the Nail

Blows to the cuticle area, including the lunula, are one of the causes of white spots on the nail. The blow jars the nail cells as the nail is being formed, and a mark is created. These marks are totally harmless, but they can be annoying if you want your nails to have an even, rosy tint. Improper manicuring techniques, which you'll learn about in later chapters, can also lead to white spots.

The *cuticle*, which is actually a thin, flexible strip of firm skin, covers most of the nail matrix, sealing the skin of the finger to the nail so that foreign objects such as bacteria can't enter the nail matrix area. It is the buildup of dry, dead cells of the cuticle adhering to the nail that can result in a hangnail— a small piece of dead skin at the side or base of the nail that is partially detached from the rest of the skin. That is why part of your natural manicure regimen will include moisturizing the cuticle and gently brushing it so that it rests firmly on the nail without actually sticking to it.

Faster! Faster! I Wish My Nails Would Grow Faster!

It is both interesting and important to understand a little about how nails grow. The finished nails that you see on your hand are composed of dead cells made up almost entirely of a protein called *keratin*. But when the production of cells begins in the nail matrix, the cells are not yet the dry material that we recognize as nails, and they contain substances other than keratin. As the cells travel from the matrix to the visible nail area, keratin production increases, and the cellular fluids dry up. The cells also become increasingly packed together. By the time the nails become visible, the cells—now all dead—have become compacted into the tough scales that form the final nail.

Nails grow continuously at a rate of about an eighth of an inch per month. It takes about four to six months to grow a totally new nail. But a number of factors can influence the speed of nail growth at any time. For instance, nails grow faster during the hormonal fluctuations of early pregnancy and during the period right before menstruation. And you may have already noticed the sudden growth spurt that occurs late each spring.

Any activity that tends to wear down the nail, such as typing or, ironically, nail biting, stimulates the rate of growth. My neighbor Annette found her nails suddenly growing very fast when she started studying massage therapy. The increased blood circulation to her fingertips stimulated growth. Possibly for this reason, nails grow faster on your right hand if you are right-handed, and vice versa.

What can *slow* nail growth? An overly stringent diet can slow nail growth as the nail bed and matrix are deprived of nutrients. And a sudden serious illness can cause a slowing in nail growth. Growth speeds up again upon recovery, leaving an indentation across the nail called a *Beau's line* as a record of the illness. While some researchers say that a Beau's line results only from very serious illness, I have noted one on my own nails after a sudden infection that involved fever. However it is produced, a Beau's line is not serious in and of itself, and will gradually travel to the tip of the nail as it grows, where the line can be filed off.

Last but not least, age affects the rate of nail growth. After the age of thirty, nail growth slows.

Nail Composition

As mentioned earlier, the nails themselves are made of layers of dead cells of a fibrous protein called keratin. Keratin is one of 50,000 proteins "custom-made" by the body from the amino acids circulating in the bloodstream. Your skin and hair are made of the same protein; in fact, as you learned earlier, the outermost layer of the skin is sometimes referred to as the keratin layer. Skin, however, is made of soft keratin, while nails and hair are made of a hard type of keratin. Nature is very thrifty, and will never invent a new protein unless it can't modify one it already has on hand. As a matter of fact, scientists have shown that nails are simply highly modified and "keratinized" cells derived from our skin.

Nail hardness stems from the presence of sulfur in an amino acid called cysteine, which binds the strands of keratin together. It is worth noting that the inherent softness or hardness of your nails is determined genetically. In other words, some people naturally have nails as hard as horse hooves, while others have nails as soft as paper. But while you may be genetically "programmed" to have soft, fragile nails, you will learn that much can be done to nourish, maintain, and strengthen them naturally.

While we're discussing the connection between the protein keratin and nail hardness, it's worth mentioning the keratin-enriched hand creams that are now sold, presumably to help strengthen nails as well as moisturize skin. While they are good moisturizers, be aware that these products will add nothing to the strength of the keratin within the nail. Keratin is produced and positioned in an orderly manner within the nail cells, so that applying a hodgepodge of cow keratin to the surface of the nail is effort in vain. You may also have heard that drinking gelatin, a brittle protein made from animal products, will strengthen your nails. Again, this is a myth; the protein in gelatin imparts no special benefits to nails.

Between the layers of the keratin are sandwiched molecules of fat and water. This gives the nail pliability and sheen. As you'll learn in Chapter 7, the fat—which, of course, is not just any old fat, but a particular type—is necessary for nail health. Therefore, if you are considering adopting a low- or no-fat diet for weight loss, you should have mercy on your nails (and skin and hair) and keep *some fat* in your diet. A strictly no-fat diet will eventually result in dull, brittle nails.

What other substances compose the nail? In addition to the sulfur already mentioned, the nail contains the minerals calcium, phosphorus, chromium, selenium, and zinc. Note that these minerals are present only in *trace* amounts. There is so little calcium present in the average nail, in fact, that scientists believe it is absorbed from outside substances such as soap. So we can debunk right now the old wives' tale about taking calcium to grow harder nails. Perhaps the old wives were confusing nails with bones, both admittedly hard substances. Calcium is important for many of your body's other structures and functions, but dermatologists agree that it is not the key to strong, healthy nails.

You may be discouraged by the fact that there's no nutritional cure-all—not calcium, not gelatin—that you can take to make your nails healthy and beautiful. But as you'll see in Chapter 7, there is plenty you *can* do from the nutritional standpoint to grow healthy nails. So don't despair!

Keeping Water at Bay

So far, we have discussed a few ways in which nails can be damaged. But we have not yet discussed one the greatest threats that everyday life poses to the nails—water.

Unlike skin, which forms a waterproof barrier to the external environment, nails are porous and can absorb water. Lots of it. In fact, your nails can absorb *20 to 25 percent of their own weight in water.* So a nail can actually increase in weight and volume as it soaks.

What happens when a nail absorbs water? The water causes the keratin fibers to swell and split apart, weakening the nail. Some skin-care experts believe that it is the repeated immersion of nails in water alternating with nail dehydration that weakens nails. Nail dehydration can occur any time the nail contains more moisture than the surrounding air. The dry air pulls moisture from the nail, causing it to contract.

Whatever the process involved, it's clear that no matter how often it may be recommended, it is inadvisable to soak your hands in warm, soapy water before a manicure. Similarly, it is unwise to relax in a long, hot bath with your fingers trailing in the water, or to do chores that expose your hands to water and detergent for any length of time.

Of course, unless you keep your hands encased in rubber gloves, it's impossible to avoid getting your nails wet sometimes. For this reason, one of the most important steps in natural nail care is *waterproofing*, a technique that you will learn in Chapter 2. Waterproofing will effectively protect your nails from the destructive cycle of waterlogging and dehydration.

A CAUTIONARY TALE

Now, I don't mean to scare anybody, but before we go on to discuss the Beautiful Hands and Nails Regimen, which is detailed in the coming chapter, let's ponder the fate of Scarlett O'Hara. As you may recall, there's a scene in *Gone With the Wind* in which Scarlett attempts to charm Rhett Butler as a means of borrowing some money from him. As part of this ruse, she must convince Rhett that everything is going well at Tara, her plantation. Scarlett first makes herself a new dress from her mother's parlor curtains, and then parades coquettishly in front of Rhett. And it almost works.

Unfortunately, after his initial delight, Rhett takes Scarlett's hands in his and looks at them—in horror! Scarlett no longer has the soft, dimpled hands he so well remembers. Instead, her hands are roughened by work and dotted with freckles. Her nails are broken and ugly. As Rhett stares at their deplorable condition, he observes that they "are not the hands of a lady," and realizes that she has been telling a lie. The result? Scarlett is forced to marry the spineless Frank Kennedy to get the money she needs!

Wow. See what can happen when you neglect your hands and nails? Disaster! Scarlett realizes too late that *she should have borrowed Aunt Pitty's gloves.*

Yes, abusing your hands can have dire, even earthshaking consequences. And as a modern woman, you don't even have the option of hiding hand and nail problems under your aunt's gloves. So if you are ever tempted to abandon your daily regimen, just think of poor Scarlett O'Hara and shudder.

Chapter 2

Your Beautiful Hands and Nails Regimen

s you learned in Chapter 1, hands and nails are delicate instruments that take a great deal of abuse each and every day. You dip them in detergents, broil them in the sun, soak them in water, and expose them to grime and germs, as well as to a variety of other substances that you probably don't want to even think about. (What *is* that coffee-colored gunk on your computer keyboard, and how did it get there?) To make matters worse, hands are the Sahara Desert of the body. With very few oil glands, they dry out easily.

Because your hands take a beating every day, they need therapy every day—just as your teeth need brushing and your face needs cleaning. That's why the four-part regimen was designed to be easily incorporated into your daily routine.

At this point, you might want to take some time and read through this entire chapter, from beginning to end. The first part of the chapter tells you about the tools and materials you'll need for your regimen. The second part details the regimen itself. After you've become familiar with what you need to buy and do, you'll want to plunge right in and start treating your hands to the simple routine that will, in time, make them as beautiful as you've always wanted them to be.

GATHERING YOUR TOOLS

The various products used in the four-part regimen are few in number, inexpensive, and easy to find in drugstores, health foods stores, and beauty supply stores. It should be noted that these are not *all* the tools and products you might want to use for hand and nail care. Later chapters will discuss other necessities—such as nail files—as well as various optional products that you might wish to add to your beauty and health arsenal. But for your basic daily regimen, the following materials are all that is needed.

❑ A Natural Bristle Nail Brush

The best nail brushes have natural bristles, with soft bristles on one side and firm bristles on the other. While nylon nail brushes are the type most commonly available, they should be avoided. Why? A look under a microscope shows that the tips of nylon bristles are as sharp and jagged as broken glass. These bristles can scratch nails and skin, doing more harm than good. Natural bristle brushes are a little harder to find, but some diligent searching in a beauty supply shop or a well-stocked drugstore should uncover just what you're looking for.

If your nails are *extremely* soft and fragile, consider using a soft-bristled toothbrush for gentle nail scrubbing. It's difficult to overdo it with such a soft-bristled brush, and you can really zero in on tiny trouble spots. Of course, you might have some explaining to do if someone comes across you brushing your nails with a toothbrush, but *c'est la vie*.

❑ Mild Liquid Castile Soap

Bottles of mild liquid castile soaps can be found in your local health foods store and in some drugstores, as well. A good, widely available brand is Dr. Bronner's Baby Castile. I recommend purchasing the smallest size available, as it is easier to grasp with slippery hands. Liquid glycerin soaps—ideally unscented—are also effective. Avoid heavily scented deodorant or medicated soaps, as these are alkaline and drying. While they may be okay for use on the rest of your body, they are not the best choice for hands and nails. What about all of the unmedicated liquid soaps that are now so widely available? These soaps are usually loaded with chemicals, and are best avoided, especially if you're prone to allergic reactions that might be triggered by fragrance or other additives.

To further soothe and soften your hands and nails, try adding a capful of pure jojoba oil to your bottle of liquid soap. Available at health foods stores, jojoba oil is actually a liquid wax that will leave behind a silkening layer of protection on your hands and nails.

If your hands are extremely dry, consider using a superfatted soap—a soap that is enriched with extra oils or fats in the form of coconut or mineral oil, lanolin, or cold cream. These soaps, which include such products as Sayman's Soap With Lanolin and Kiss My Face soap with olive oil, will add that extra bit of moisturizing that your hands may need. During the very coldest winter months, when the air outdoors is frigid and the air indoors is dried by central heating, you may be plagued by bleeding and cracking skin on your hands and around your nails. If so, consider "washing" your hands with only a light-textured hand lotion for a day or two—just until your hands can begin to heal. When you start using soap and water again, be sure to dry your hands very thoroughly afterwards and to apply a moisturizer immediately.

❑ A Nail Protector

Nail protector is my term for any waterproof coating that seals moisture into the nail and repels water and dirt. Waxy lip balms such as Chap Stick perform this function perfectly. I know that it may seem strange to suggest using a lip balm on nails instead of lips, but these products work so well that you couldn't invent anything better if you tried. They are wonderful nail waterproofers and are inexpensive, too.

To afford your nails the greatest protection possible, use a lip balm that contains a sunscreen. Nails are as susceptible to sun damage as any other part of your body, so a sunscreen-enriched lip balm is a great choice. Lip balms that contain vitamin E, panthenol, and botanicals such as aloe vera are also fine for nails. Waxy lip balms can be found in any drugstore, of course, but check your local health foods store, as well.

One last nail protector note: Be sure that the lip balm you purchase is *waxy* in consistency. Some of the newer products are more oily than waxy. While this makes them more pleasant to use on lips, it's the wax you need to waterproof your nails.

❏ A Nail Nourisher

Nighttime is the perfect opportunity to replenish the moisture your nails and cuticles lose during the day. And any one of a number of products—including, but not limited to, petroleum jelly, wheat germ oil, vitamin E oil, lanolin, Carmex lip balm, A and D Ointment, and homemade Nail Butter (see page 36)—can perform this job beautifully. All of these products have one thing in common: They are viscous in consistency. This means that they are too thick to flow, or, at least, that they don't flow quickly. Rather, they stick to the nail and tend to accumulate in the groove of the cuticle. So when you wake up in the morning, the nail nourisher will still be nourishing your nails, and won't be on the bed sheets. This is why just any old oil—for instance, olive oil, which is so often recommended for this purpose—isn't optimal for nighttime use.

Which nail nourisher is best for you? To a degree, you can let your own preferences be your guide. You may simply like using one product better than another. And if that product works for you, by all means, keep using it.

Sometimes, though, specific problems make the use of a specific product more appropriate. For instance, vitamin E oil is your best choice if you tend to have hangnails, especially inflamed hangnails. Research has shown that the oil actually speeds the healing of fresh wounds. Just pierce a vitamin E capsule with a pin, and squeeze out a drop of oil onto the nail and cuticle area. I have found that one capsule contains enough oil for three or four days. Of all the nail nourishers, vitamin E oil is among the most viscous. This means that it will cling to your nails even if you toss and turn at night. Do be aware, though, that vitamin E does cause some people to have an allergic reaction. For this reason, it's wise to try just a dab on one or two nails for a few nights before using it on all your nails. If you are allergic, you'll soon find out. Your skin will become reddened and itchy.

Wheat germ oil—which, like vitamin E, is available in capsules—is another option. This oil contains vitamin A, another skin and nail vitamin, as well as vitamin E. It also contains a substance called octacosanol, which appears to enhance the antioxidant actions of vitamins A and E. Although wheat germ oil is a bit more difficult to find than vitamin E, it's worth the search.

Petroleum jelly is especially good for moisturizing dehydrated nails and cuticles. Research has shown that a layer of petroleum jelly forms what is called an *occlusive barrier* over the nails and cuticles. This is a film that prevents drying air from getting into the cuticle, and prevents moisture from escaping. In addition, the fats in the jelly actually penetrate the surface layers of the skin and nails. Keep in mind, though, that although this product is great for hands and nails, it should probably not be used elsewhere on your body, where its occlusive nature could contribute to skin breakouts.

If you have splitting nails and cracked fingertips—serious problems, in other words—pure lanolin make a great nail nourisher. Also known as wool fat, lanolin does tend to be sticky, though, and so is a bit trickier to use than the other nourishers. Just crumple a tissue and catch a dab of the lanolin on it. Then apply the dab to the nail. Buy your lanolin in the smallest available container, as it's used in only tiny amounts. I'm still working my way through a one-pound jar of lanolin that I purchased six years ago!

Allergic to wool? Lanolin may or may not cause a problem for you. Some people are allergic to wool, but have no problem with lanolin. (I'm one of those people, actually.) In later chapters, we'll use lanolin in a winter hand treatment. Otherwise, though, I don't recommend using this product as an overall hand moisturizer, as this definitely would cause problems for allergic individuals.

❑ Daytime Hand Cream or Lotion

Hand creams and lotions are a basic and invaluable hand and nail care tool. You'll want to apply a cream or lotion as part of your morning routine, and reapply it throughout the day, especially after you wash your hands or otherwise immerse them in water. (A different type of hand cream, best for nighttime use, is discussed later in the chapter.)

In my experience, homemade hand creams and lotions are too heavy and greasy for daytime use. And the best daily hand cream contains a sunscreen, an ingredient that would be difficult for you to locate and purchase. So exactly what should you look for in a cream or lotion? First, you'll want a product with an SPF (sun protection factor) of 15 or higher. Hand creams that contain sunscreen protect your skin from the aging effects of the sun's rays, and so block the development of brown spots on the backs of the hands. And you *do* want to prevent those spots.

Second, look for a cream or lotion that is thick and creamy in consistency. Thin-textured, drippy moisturizers, often very inexpensive because they contain a lot of water, may be easier to apply than their thicker counterparts, but as their water content evaporates, your skin is left with only a skimpy protective coat. Creamy lotions are more concentrated, and contain more of the ingredients that your skin needs.

Finally, as unscientific as it may sound, you'll want a product whose fragrance and consistency you find pleasing. If you really, really like a lotion, you'll use it a lot. If you don't, you won't. I use a lotion with a faint lavender-herbal scent that smells clean to me. You might prefer something with a more traditional floral scent, or perhaps something with no scent at all.

As hand lotions that contain sunscreen are not common (yet!), look among the sunscreens and all-purpose moisturizers and body lotions for your daytime hand lotion. Johnson & Johnson's Dual Purpose Treatment Moisturizer with an SPF of 15 is a nice unscented, light-textured lotion. Nivea also has some good lotions that contain sunscreen. Neutrogena's New Hands also has a sunscreen, although because it is formulated specifically for the back of the hand, this product may seem too heavy for use on your entire hand. Also look for sunscreens whose textures are similar to that of hand creams. While some sunscreens are too greasy for this purpose, the ingredients and consistency of certain products are nearly identical to those of some hand lotions! Coppertone sunscreens for children are quite nice for hands. These products have a mild scent—not the "sun and sand" aroma of so many sunscreens—and come in a range of sun protection factors.

If most hand creams seem too greasy for you, try a lotion like Lac-Hydrin Five from Westwood-Squibb Pharmaceuticals. This product has a velvety texture that's distinctly different from that of most lotions, and it may do the trick for you. Since it doesn't contain a sunscreen, though, you will still need a separate sunscreen for the backs of your hands.

❏ **Nighttime Hand Cream**

Just before going to bed, and after you apply your nail nourisher, you'll want to smooth some cream onto your hands. While you want to avoid greasy creams during the day, bedtime is a great opportunity to use a rich commercial cream or, perhaps, a homemade cream, such as my Hand Butter (page 37). The inexpensive, vitamin-enriched creams often sold as night creams or face creams are great for this use. Also good are creams containing alpha-hydroxy acids.

❏ **"White" Iodine**

Also called *iodides tincture* or *decolorized iodine*, white iodine

Formulas for Beautiful Hands and Nails

As you'll learn throughout this book, drugstores, health foods stores, and beauty supply shops offer a variety of products that can help you heal your hands and nails and, later, maintain their health. But sometimes you may want to whip up something in your own kitchen as a special treat for your hands. These homemade products are easy to make and a delight to use. Most important, you'll have the satisfaction of knowing that these products contain simple, gentle, *natural* ingredients that are truly good for your hands and nails.

Most of the ingredients for the formulas you'll find in this book can be purchased at local stores. Check your health foods store for the liquid lecithin and apricot kernel oil. Lanolin and glycerin are available at most drugstores. Beeswax is often available in health foods stores and hobby stores. If any of the ingredients called for cannot be found locally, however, you can easily order them from the suppliers found in the Resource List on page 133.

Plastic jars sold to carry cosmetics during travel are ideal for storing these products, as are the small recycled jars from cosmetic samples. Small wide-mouthed jars work, too. If you decide to continue making your own beauty products—and the next chapter contains a few more ideas—you'll find yourself saving containers that are appropriate for this purpose.

Nail Butter

Here's a simple recipe for your very own homemade nail nourisher. You'll see why it's called Nail Butter when you make it. It's full of good things for your nails, and its buttery texture makes it a pleasure to use. You can also use this product as a lip gloss.

Yield: 1/3 cup

2 tablespoons liquid lecithin
2 tablespoons apricot kernel oil
1 tablespoon lanolin
1/4 ounce white beeswax, chipped*
Contents of 1 vitamin E capsule

*Cut a 1-ounce cylinder or cube of beeswax into four equal parts to get 1/4 ounce.

1. Place all of the ingredients in a heatproof glass measuring cup. Then place the cup in a saucepan containing an inch of water, and place over low heat.

2. Heat, occasionally stirring with the tip of a dinner knife, for about 5 minutes, or until the ingredients have melted. Pour the mixture into a small container, and allow to cool to room temperature. Cover and store at room temperature, using as desired.

Hand Butter

This kissing cousin of Nail Butter is lighter, fluffier, and more "whipped" in texture. Thick and rich, it is perfect for use as a night-time hand cream. You can customize Hand Butter by adding a little vitamin E and vitamin A oil from capsules, or even a little jojoba oil.

Yield: about ½ cup

¼ cup apricot kernel oil
¼ ounce white beeswax, chipped*
1 teaspoon lanolin
1 teaspoon liquid lecithin
1 tablespoon glycerin

*Cut a 1-ounce cylinder or cube of beeswax into four equal parts to get ¼ ounce.

1. Place all of the ingredients except for the glycerin in a heatproof glass measuring cup. Then place the cup in a saucepan containing an inch of water, and place over low heat.

2. Heat, occasionally stirring with the tip of a dinner knife, for about 5 minutes, or until the ingredients have melted.

3. Allow the mixture to cool to room temperature. Stir in the glycerin, continuing to stir for a few moments until the mixture has a "whipped" texture.

4. Transfer the mixture to a container and cover. Store at room temperature, using as desired.

is an effective and inexpensive antiseptic. This product is not a *must* item, but should be purchased if you have a problem with hangnails or torn cuticles. Look for it in the first aid aisle, next to the Mercurochrome and other antiseptics.

TAKING THE FIRST STEP

You've now gathered your "tools" together, and you're ready to begin your four-part program. First, though, you'll want to prepare your nails so that they can receive the greatest benefit from the regimen.

To begin, if you are wearing nail polish, it's time to remove it—at least temporarily. Later, you can decide whether you want to continue wearing polish. Now your nails need to be free of polishes and hardeners so that they can breathe and soak up the moisture and nourishment provided by the treatment.

Remove the polish as thoroughly as possible; then wash and rinse your hands carefully to rid them of any traces of the polish remover. If your nails have been stained by years of polish use, just leave the stains there for the time being. They'll gradually wear away. Using more nail polish remover could cause severe drying.

Now, you will want to use a sharp nail clipper to clip your nails short. Actually, you may not *want* to do this, but think of it as putting your nails in the hospital for rest and rehabilitation. Clipping the nails short jettisons many old nail problems—the chips, the splits, and the dried-out, yellowed nail tips. It's time for a fresh start. In the future, you won't use a nail clipper at all. But for now, it's the quickest way to get your nails short and fairly equal in length. How short is short? Make your nails as short as you can tolerate, with the white nail tip no more than an eighth of an inch in length. If you have a nail (or nails) that is chewed to the quick, just clip the other nails short. In time, the problem nail will catch up.

Now, as best you can, lightly smooth any rough or uneven spots, preferably with the help of a metal nail file coated with diamond or sapphire dust. This type of file, available wherever nail-care products are sold, is easy on your nails, as gem dusts are very fine, hard abrasives. If you prefer to use cardboard files (emery boards), buy a good-quality file, and be prepared to replace it often, as these files wear out quite quickly. I have found that very inexpensive emery boards are unevenly coated with a rather coarse abrasive. You might as well use sandpaper on your nails! So take the time to find a high-quality product. (See Chapter 4 for more information on nail files.)

Remember that in the days to come, you'll be doing more nail filing, shaping, and smoothing. But for now, you want to focus on simply returning your nails to health.

THE FOUR-PART REGIMEN

Now that you have gathered your supplies and prepared the ground, so to speak, you're ready to start treating your hands and nails to the tender loving care they deserve. I think you'll love the big difference this regimen will make.

The Beautiful Hands and Nails Regimen consists of four simple steps to be performed daily. It is the foundation for having hands and nails with a meticulously clean, well-cared-for appearance.

The first step in the regimen is a deep nail cleaning that is performed each morning with a nail brush, mild soap, and water. This not only cleans the nails, but removes dead skin cells from the cuticles, as well. Nothing unusual so far, right?

The second step, which *is* a bit unusual, is a morning application of a waxy nail protector that seals moisture into the nails during the day. This counteracts fluctuations in nail hydration, the source of so many nail problems.

The third step, which is really more of an ongoing process than a step, is to intensively moisturize your hands. This is performed first as part of the morning ritual, and then on a continual basis throughout the day to keep your hands hydrated and to protect them from the sun. Your new motto should be: *Never have naked hands!*

The final step, performed in the evening before going to bed, is to apply a nail nourisher that penetrates the nails, moisturizing and conditioning them overnight.

Each morning, the cycle should begin again as you brush

away the previous night's nail nourisher with soap and water. Simple? Yes, very. Effective? Yes . . . especially when it's done *every day.* I like to think of this regimen as daily therapy for your hands and nails. So let's begin.

Step 1: Brushing Your Nails

Nail brushing, an essential part of nail care, can make a huge difference in nail and cuticle appearance. First, brushing removes accumulated dirt and grime from the nails and fingertips. Second, it removes excess dead skin cells from the cuticles, helping to prevent hangnails. Third, brushing under the nails shapes the nail bed into a pretty, evenly rounded arc. And last, but just as important, brushing stimulates the circulation of blood to the nail beds, promoting nail health.

To brush your nails, have at hand your nail brush and liquid soap. Wet the brush with warm water, and apply a small amount of soap—about the size of a dime—to the soft bristle side. Then lightly brush the nails of both hands, moving the brush back and forth across the width of the nail. This initial brushing allows the soap to suds up, and starts softening the cuticles.

When a generous amount of suds has formed, turn the brush over and, using the firm bristles, again brush back and forth across the nail. Because these side areas are where hangnails often form, they benefit from special attention. If you have any hangnails or inflamed areas, skip over them, but do all of the other nails as best you can. Repeat this process for each nail.

Try to take a little extra time to brush the nails of your little fingers, as they are usually neglected, and as a result, can develop hard, overgrown cuticles. In addition, if you compare the little fingers of both hands, you may find that one nail is a lot bigger than the other. Right-handed people, for instance, often have larger nails on their right hands, and left-handed people, on their left hands. For some reason, this tendency is most noticeable on the little fingers. In the great scheme of things, this certainly isn't the end of the world, but in the name of nail harmony, you might want to give the smaller nail a bit of extra brushing, as this can enlarge the nail surface.

When the sides of all the nails have been brushed, turn your hand over and brush back and forth under your nails using the firm bristles. Be gentle but thorough.

As you brush—and, really, in all nail care procedures—please aim to be as gentle as possible with your nails. I purposely haven't called this step nail scrubbing, as *scrubbing* sounds a bit too much like scouring floors or preparing for a surgical procedure. The mild sudsing action of the liquid castile or glycerin soap, combined with careful brushing with the natural bristle brush, will gently but thoroughly deep clean your nails as the days go by.

After a few days of brushing, you may notice small fragments of loosened dead skin peeling away from the cuticles. If so, fine. It's this dead, dried cuticle skin that is the breeding ground for hangnails. I don't know about you, but I'm glad to see it go.

Although I have said that your nails should be brushed every morning, this is actually necessary only for the first week or two. Beyond this point, daily brushing may be too harsh and drying for some extremely soft, fragile nails, so you'll need to evaluate how often you should brush. Signs of overbrushing may include tenderness of the cuticle and nail drying. Or little splits may occur on the surface of the nail. If your nails are very soft and your overall skin type sensitive, you may want to brush only two or three times a week. If in doubt, *it is always better to underdo than overdo.*

Avoiding Chapped Hands and Nails

When you're finished brushing the nails on both hands, rinse them well, and dry them thoroughly with a soft clean towel. Thorough drying can help to prevent the hands—and the nails—from becoming chapped. Did you know that your *nails* can become chapped? It's true. If damp nails are exposed to dry air, the air rapidly pulls the moisture out of them, causing a weakening in the nail structure as well as a dull-looking nail surface. By thoroughly drying both hands, you can prevent this from occurring.

Treating Hangnails

Once your nails have been brushed and thoroughly dried, it's time to apply white iodine to any hangnails or torn, inflamed areas of the cuticle, if you have them. Yes, this can sting a little, but it will speed up the drying and healing of any inflammation.

If you have a very new and really horrendous hangnail—one that has torn deeply into the skin—wash that area with antibacterial soap and water, but wait a day before applying the iodine. If you use it right away, it might sting a lot. (For an effective strategy for healing badly torn hangnails, see page 58.)

Step 2: Protecting Your Nails

As soon as you have finished brushing and drying your nails, apply your nail protector. This will seal the moisture into your nails and prevent dehydration.

To apply the nail protector, first apply a small amount of lip balm to the top surface of each nail. Then curl over the fingers of that hand and cradle it in the other hand. This will allow you to use the thumb of the second hand to massage the protector into your nails and cuticles. Do be sure to include the cuticle, as some nail problems actually originate from neglected cuticles. Dried and roughened cuticles can become a magnet for nervous picking and biting, and pretty soon, both your cuticles and your nails can be in trouble. Use gentle pressure, as this will not only spread the protector, but also give each fingertip a little circulation-boosting massage.

At first, you may be a bit hesitant about using a nail protector, wondering if it won't be greasy. Don't worry. Using a very small amount of your chosen nail protector on each nail will yield an attractive sheen without greasiness. If you've used too much, just tissue off the excess. At this point, I hope, you'll start looking among the many lip balms available and experimenting with them. For instance, there are cherry-flavored lip balms and "lip toned" balms that can add a touch of color to your nails. Lip balms are inexpensive, so you can afford to buy a bunch and stash them in your purse, your coat pocket, and your desk drawer at work, as well as in your bathroom at home. And, of course, there's nothing wrong with using them on your lips, too!

Later in the day, you may have to reapply your nail protector, just as you might reapply lipstick. To do this on the run, just curl over the fingers of one hand and apply a streak of the lip balm over four fingers at once, and then over the thumb. Briefly rub the balm in. Then do the other hand.

Step 3: Protecting Your Hands

After you brush and protect your nails, it will be time to protect your hands. Apply your chosen hand cream or lotion liberally, rubbing it in well all over your hands. Don't forget your knuckles, a much-neglected area of the body. The crevices in the skin of the knuckles are thin so that you can easily bend your fingers. This makes knuckles especially vulnerable to chapping.

On cold winter's days, especially, spend a little extra time massaging the cream or lotion into your skin—it could prevent bleeding and cracking. (If your hands *do* bleed and crack, try massaging in a little vitamin E or wheat germ oil.) If you find that you've used too much cream—and this does happen—rub the excess into your elbows, another thirsty area of your body. They'll thank you for it.

Apply your cream or lotion frequently during the day. One of the secrets to beautiful hands is to keep them protected from the sun with a sunscreen and constantly moisturized, all day and every day. I know—ho hum. It's not always easy to keep at it. But the dry, delicate skin of your hands, especially the vulnerable backs, needs protection every second.

Keep containers of your hand lotion dotted about the house

at every sink so that you will be encouraged to apply it every time you wash your hands. For home use, I strongly recommend hand cream that comes in a pump dispenser, as this makes it easier to use. Then keep tubes of lotion in your purse, in your desk at work, and in the glove compartment of your car. Remember: *It is impossible to overmoisturize your hands.*

Step 4: Nourishing Your Nails

Now we come to the evening, and to the end of the four-part regimen of daily hand and nail care. During the day, your nails have been assaulted by soaps, detergents, the drying rays of the sun, pollution—you name it. So you need to repair the damage with a good nail nourisher.

After you've showered, bathed, or washed your hands for the last time before getting into bed, apply a tiny dab of one of the nail nourishers described on page 32 to each nail. Then rub in the nourisher. For the first two weeks of the program, do this very carefully, taking time to massage the nourisher well into both the nails *and* the cuticles. Afterwards—once your hands and nails have begun to improve—you can be a bit more casual. When you're in a hurry, simply apply some nourisher over all your nails at once, and, holding your fingers together, massage them all at the same time.

After you apply the nail nourisher to your nails, it's a good idea to smooth some rich cream onto your hands. This is the time to use your nighttime hand cream. (See page 35.) Take the time to massage as much of the cream into your hands as you can to moisturize and rejuvenate your skin as you sleep.

THE KEY TO BEAUTIFUL HANDS AND NAILS

So there you have it—the four basic steps to getting and maintaining pretty hands and nails. I can't emphasize enough the importance of making this regimen a daily habit. Because your hands and nails are so low in natural moisture, if not properly cared for, they can very quickly go from being wonderful in appearance to being really horrible.

In the coming chapters, you'll learn about additional hand and nail care procedures. But this four-part regimen is the *minimum* necessary to return your hands and nails to good health and to protect them from daily wear and tear.

Chapter 3

Gentle Cuticle Care for Beautiful Nails

You might wonder if a whole chapter devoted to cuticle care isn't a bit excessive, but I really believe that healthy cuticles are the secret to beautiful, healthy nails. For this reason, cuticle care is more important than you think. Certainly, dry, hard, roughened cuticles are often the magnet for nervous picking and biting. Smooth cuticles stymie this nervous behavior, giving nails a chance to grow unimpeded. And, of course, well-cared-for, attractively shaped cuticles form beautiful frames for your nails. So any time spent on cuticle care is time well spent!

Regular and gentle nail brushing and moisturizing—both a part of your Beautiful Hands and Nails Regimen—will help keep cuticles free of excess dead skin cells. But sometimes cuticles need extra help. As you know, drugstores and beauty supply stores offer many commercial products designed to eliminate unsightly cuticles. But commercial cuticle removers are caustic alkali-based compounds that can badly irritate any hangnails you may have, possibly leading to cuticle infection. If this sounds like something you want to avoid, you'll be glad to know that there are plenty of *natural* ways to smooth, soothe, and heal cuticles.

In this chapter, you'll learn about daily habits—habits that can be easily made a part of your four-step regimen—that can help shape your cuticles. You'll also learn about natural substances, from cornmeal to lavender oil to grapefruit peel, that can smooth and soften problem cuticles. A helpful inset will let you know about some cuticle don'ts—cuticle care techniques that can actually *harm* your nails. And, finally, you'll learn about the best and fastest way to heal those bothersome hangnails.

SHAPING YOUR CUTICLES

In Chapter 2, I discussed the importance of daily nail brushing. This practice keeps the cuticles free of excess dead skin cells, and prevents the cuticle from adhering to the nail, a situation that can lead to hangnails. Truly the cornerstone of cuticle care, daily brushing can eliminate and prevent many problems.

To further help improve the appearance of your cuticles, you might want to gently push them back after brushing the nails as part of your daily routine. A great tool for this job is a manicure implement called a *cuticle trimmer.* Sold wherever nail-care tools are found, the cuticle trimmer has two ends. One end is wedge-shaped and used to push back the cuticle, preventing it from adhering to your nail. The other end— which is a tiny stainless steel V-shaped trimming edge—is used to skim off rough, dry cuticle skin.

To shape your cuticles, first use the wedge-shaped end to gently and evenly push the cuticle back to yield a rounded shape. (See Figure 3.1.) Pay special attention to the sides of the nail.

Once the cuticles are pushed back, it's time to use the trimmer end. Be sure to trim only those cuticles that are healthy and free of hangnails. If you do have hangnails or tender or raw cuticles, wait until they are completely healed before using the trimmer. Then simply position the trimmer at one end of a cuticle, holding it almost parallel to the nail and just slightly angled down into the cuticle, with its prongs facing

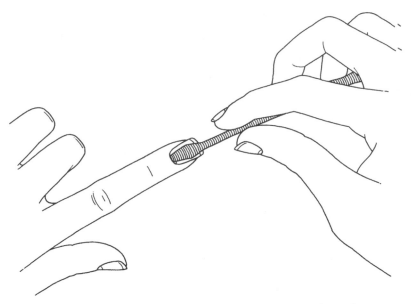

Use the wedge-shaped end of the trimmer to gently push
the cuticle back into a rounded shape.

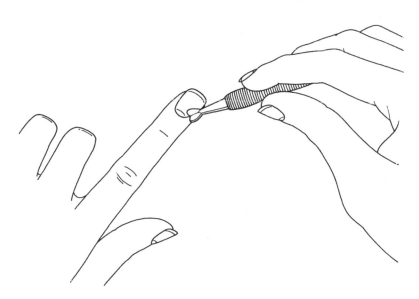

With the prongs facing upward and the trimmer held almost
parallel to the nail, use the V-shaped end to gently skim off
the dead skin of the cuticle ridge.

Figure 3.1 Using a Cuticle Trimmer

upward. The trimmer works by skimming off dead skin from the cuticle edge, not by digging or scooping into it. As you move the trimmer along the cuticle edge, press down very lightly into the cuticle. You will see the dead skin being trimmed off.

The trimmer can yield smooth cuticles so quickly and neatly that you may be tempted to try to trim off every little bit of dead skin. To avoid injury to the cuticle, though, I advise using the trimmer only once a week. Daily nail brushing, daily moisturizing, and use of some of the cuticle smoothers described in the next few pages are the best ways to keep cuticles smooth, soft, and pliable on a daily basis.

If you choose not to use a cuticle trimmer, or if you are unable to locate one, you can push back and shape your cuticles with the use of a soft towel. While a towel is not quite as effective as the specially designed implement—and, of course, does not have a trimming edge—it will work. Try to use it after you've taken a bath or finished brushing your nails, as your cuticles will then be a bit softer than usual.

After pushing back your cuticles and trimming them as necessary, you may find that some of the dead skin of the cuticle has adhered to the nail. A manicure implement called a *hindostone* can be used to remove the dead skin. Like cuticle trimmers, hindostones are sold with other nail-care products, usually among the nail files. Sometimes called stone files, they are made of a slightly abrasive stone. (See Chapter 4 for more about this and other nail files.) To use, lightly moisten the tip of the hindostone with water, and gently rub the moistened tip over the adhering cuticle tissue. If all of the dead skin doesn't come off after ten or fifteen seconds of gentle rubbing, stop, and try again a few days later. As with many aspects of nail care, a little gentle persistence is better than risking injury to the nail. The daily nail brushing will also work to remove this dead skin.

After using the cuticle trimmer or hindostone, massage a little cuticle salve or nail protector into the cuticle and nail. This will smooth and moisturize the cuticle, helping it to look its best.

Avoiding the Pitfalls of Cuticle Care

As you'll learn throughout this chapter, there is much you can do to shape, smooth, and heal problem cuticles. But there are also some very common practices that can actually *harm* your cuticles. Here are a few practices you'll want to avoid.

❑ Do not use manicure scissors, nail clippers, or nail nippers to trim the cuticle ridge. These powerful implements can easily cut into the living tissue of the cuticle, allowing bacteria to enter the area, and possibly leading to infection. However, when properly used, a cuticle trimmer is a safe means of trimming dry, dead skin from the cuticle ridge. (See page 48 for details.) And if there are any dead bits of skin protruding from the cuticle—hangnails, in other words—you may carefully cut them off with nail clippers. These bits of skin can snag in clothes or other objects, causing a tear in the cuticle. Whether using a cuticle trimmer or removing a hangnail, just be sure to avoid cutting the living tissue.

❑ Never use a sharp-tipped manicure implement to dig under the cuticle in an effort to lift it off the nail. This can damage the matrix, the area where the new nail is formed, causing the nail to grow in with lines, ridges, or white spots. Be assured that it's persistent, gentle care that yields smooth cuticles and healthy nails. There really is no substitute!

❑ I've said it before, but it bears repeating—do not approach cuticle care or any nail care with too much vigor! Again, a too-enthusiastic approach can cause more problems than it solves. Be gentle and have patience.

Once you get into a nail-care routine, you will probably find yourself shaping your cuticles this way every week or so. A caution is in order, however. Don't be too enthusiastic when pushing back or trimming your cuticles! It is better to do this too little than too much. Cuticles form a shield against the invasion of bacteria and other microbes, preventing the organisms from entering the matrix—the area that generates new nail growth. Harming this shield can lead to problems such as infection. In addition, vigorous pushing may cause crosswise ridges, bumps, or indentations in the nail surface. These bumps and ridges may become visible weeks later, leaving you to wonder what caused them. Dermatologists say that some of the nail problems they see are actually the result of *overgrooming*, not of negligence. So be gentle!

How long will it take to develop really smooth cuticles? Considering that it took months, perhaps even years, for dead skin cells to build up on your cuticles, you can't realistically expect any hardened skin to disappear overnight. With regular brushing, moisturizing, and shaping, though, you'll remove a few more layers of dead cells every day. And within three weeks or so, you should see a dramatic improvement. But the timetable all depends on the initial condition of your cuticles.

SMOOTHING YOUR CUTICLES

Years of chemical treatments or just plain neglect can leave you with thick, dry, hard cuticles. While the Beautiful Hands and Nails Regimen will steadily slough away any unsightly dead cuticle skin, there are natural ways to exfoliate more quickly, revealing smooth, healthy looking cuticles. Use the following smoothers along with your four-part regimen whenever you feel that your cuticles need special attention— for instance, at summer's end, when your hands and nails show signs of too much exposure to sun and wind.

When using even these natural treatments, a word of caution is advisable. Use exfoliants only on the nail and cuticle areas, or on calluses found on the sides of the fingers. Even gentle exfoliants like these should never be used on the back of the hand, a dry area that can be easily harmed.

Cornmeal Cuticle Smoother

The Cornmeal Cuticle Smoother will allow you to exfoliate your cuticles gently, without harsh chemical cuticle removers and without stinging or burning. I was really surprised by how effective this treatment is—and how good it feels. Even if you have a hangnail or two, this treatment is appropriate. Just skip over the hangnail and massage the rest of the cuticle.

To use Cornmeal Cuticle Smoother, simply moisten your fingertips with water and dip them into a teaspoon or so of white or yellow cornmeal. (I keep a supply of organic cornmeal in a small covered plastic bowl by the bathroom sink.) Rub and massage the cornmeal thoroughly into the cuticles. Then rinse carefully. You may want to use a nail brush to make sure that all the particles of cornmeal are removed. Finally, use a clean, rough terry cloth towel to dry each nail. Use this treatment as often as once a week.

Violet-Scented Cuticle Smoother

A further refinement of the Cornmeal Cuticle Smoother is the Violet-Scented Cuticle Smoother. To make it, simply add about one part orris root powder to about two parts white cornmeal. Orris root powder is made from the root of a special iris, and can be found in well-stocked health foods stores. If you find only whole dried orris root, simply process it in your blender along with the cornmeal to get it to the proper consistency. The powder will lend a violet scent to the mixture, making it more like a cosmetic and less like a foodstuff. Use it as you would use the Cornmeal Cuticle Smoother.

MOISTURIZING AND HEALING YOUR CUTICLES

While the exfoliants just mentioned will help gently slough away any dead skin, they won't necessarily soothe and heal the remaining cuticle. The following treatments, however, can soften, moisturize, and, in many cases, heal cuticles that have become dry, hard, rough, and split. Each of these treatments is slightly different, though, so read the descriptions carefully. You'll want to choose the remedy that will suit your problem.

As usual, I urge caution in the use of even these natural

beauty aids. The longer I study and use nail and cuticle care, the more I am convinced that the cuticle area must be handled very carefully to prevent the formation of white spots, nail ridges, or tiny dark lines in the nail. So massage these treatments in *gently*, working on each individual finger for only a short time. Do not apply any treatment with too much vigor.

Lavender Cuticle Soother

Aromatherapy oils, often called essential oils, are extracted from aromatic plants and used for cosmetic and medicinal purposes. Despite claims to the contrary, I haven't found that any essential oil can actually stimulate nail growth. But there are a number of oils that can soften roughened cuticles, as well as heal any small tears.

When you use aromatherapy oils, keep in mind that they are very concentrated, and that some can actually irritate the skin when used undiluted. Therefore, unless I specify otherwise, you'll want to add a number of drops to a mild "carrier" oil, such as wheat germ, sweet almond, jojoba, apricot kernel, or grapeseed oil.

A number of aromatherapy oils can be used to soothe and heal rough and ragged cuticles. You might want to try chamomile, carrot, tea tree, patchouli, rose, eucalyptus, myrrh, and geranium oils. My own favorite is lavender oil. In addition to being moderately priced and clean smelling, lavender has been shown to have both antibacterial and anti-fungal properties—definite benefits when you're dealing with the cuticle and nail. It is also soothing, and can help heal inflamed hangnails.

To make Lavender Cuticle Soother, simply add a few drops of the lavender oil to a teaspoon of wheat germ oil. If desired, also add a few drops of tea tree oil, another known infection fighter and wound healer. You might want to make a little more of this mixture than is needed for a single application, and store it in a small glass jar. It will stay fresh for several weeks.

To use Lavender Cuticle Soother, apply a tiny drop to the

cuticle area of each nail, and massage it in gently. You do not have to rub in the entire drop, as any residue will sink in with time. Use this treatment as often as desired.

Fresh Grapefruit Oil Soother

The next time you have grapefruit for breakfast, save a shard of the peel for a vitamin-packed cuticle treatment. While this may sound a little crazy, it works. The white pithy part of the peel is loaded with fresh grapefruit oil. This, in turn, contains vitamin C and food compounds called *phytochemicals*, vitamin-like plant compounds with antioxidant properties. While I have no scientific evidence that these nutrients soften cuticles, my own experience has shown that grapefruit peel smoothes the cuticle and helps to heal any small abrasions or tears. It also cleans and smoothes calluses.

To benefit from the wonderful effects of grapefruit oil, just take a small fragment of the peel and gently rub the white inner portion over both your cuticles and nails. For best results, use fresh peel for each treatment, as once the peel is removed from the grapefruit, the oils can break down quickly. Use this treatment as often as desired.

Warm Apricot Kernel Oil Cuticle Softener

If your cuticles seem especially dry and hard, give them a special treat by massaging them with warm apricot kernel oil. Easy to find at most well-stocked health foods stores, this oil seems to have an especially healing and beneficial quality, as though the warmth of the sun is captured in the oil.

To prepare the treatment, place a teaspoon of the oil in a small glass dish, and warm in a microwave for about 20 seconds. If using a conventional stovetop, place the oil in a small saucepan over low heat just until warm.

To use Warm Apricot Oil Cuticle Softener, apply a tiny drop to the cuticle area of each nail, and massage it in gently. This treatment is so gentle that you may use it each and every day.

~ 55 ~

Formulas for Smooth, Supple Cuticles

Throughout this chapter, you've learned about the many widely available products, from cornmeal to castor oil, that can help you gently exfoliate, soothe, and heal problem cuticles. Some of these remedies can be used as is. Others need only be heated briefly before use. At some point, though, you might want to try making a slightly more sophisticated product for use on your cuticles. The following formulas will delight you with the ease with which they can be prepared, as well as the wonderful things they'll do for your cuticles.

Like the ingredients used in the homemade hand- and nail-care products presented in Chapter 2, most of the ingredients listed below are readily available at local sources. Look for apricot kernel oil in your health foods store, and lanolin in your local drugstore. Any ingredient that you cannot locate can be ordered by mail from the suppliers found in the Resource List on page 133.

Apricot Oil–Lanolin Cuticle Salve

This buttery salve combines the healing benefits of apricot kernel oil with the rich emollient qualities of lanolin. Just rub a tiny dab into your cuticles every day or whenever you feel that your cuticles need an extra bit of TLC.

Yield: 2½ teaspoons

½ teaspoon apricot kernel oil
2 teaspoons lanolin
1 drop essential oil of your choice (optional)

1. Place the apricot kernel oil and lanolin in a heatproof cup or bowl. (If desired, use the container you will store the mixture in, as long as it's heatproof. A ½-ounce jar is perfect.) Then place the container in a saucepan containing an inch of water, and place over low heat.

2. Heat, occasionally stirring with the tip of a dinner knife, until the lanolin melts. At this point, if desired, stir in a drop of essential oil, such as lavender oil.

3. Allow the mixture to cool to room temperature, stirring several times during cooling. Cover and store at room temperature, using as desired.

Calendula Cuticle Salve

Calendula flowers contain carotenoids, vitamin-like substances that help skin cells heal and regenerate. When steeped in petroleum jelly, a wonderful healing ointment is created—one that is not only great on ragged cuticles, but also works as a nail nourisher. You will find this salve especially helpful if you suffer from inflamed hangnails, or if your nails are so bitten down that they have become sore.

You can order calendula flowers from mail order firms that specialize in dried herbs and botanicals. You may also be able to find them at a well-stocked health foods store. Of course, if you have a garden, you can easily grow the flowers yourself.

Yield: ½ cup

½ cup dried calendula flowers (1 ounce)
4-ounce jar petroleum jelly

1. Place the flowers in a 1-cup glass bowl, and add the petroleum jelly. Place the bowl in a sturdy saucepan containing an inch of water. (Do not attempt to make this salve directly over the heat.)

2. Place the saucepan over low heat until the jelly melts, stirring several times during the melting process. Remove the mixture from the heat, cover, and allow to steep overnight.

3. The next day, drain off any fluid that has accumulated on the jelly. Place over low heat, and allow to melt, stirring occasionally.

4. Pour the hot mixture through a clean nylon stocking or other strainer, straining it into a covered jar. (You can use the original petroleum jelly jar.) Press the mixture with a spoon to extract all of the salve.

5. Allow to cool to room temperature, cover, and store at room temperature, using as desired.

Variation

To make Clover Cuticle Salve, simply follow the directions for Calendula Cuticle Salve, but substitute red clover blossoms for the calendula. Clover blossoms pop up on lawns in early and mid-summer. You don't have to let the blossoms dry completely—just let them wilt to concentrate the plant material a bit. Red clover blossoms have long been used to treat skin problems such as sores, rashes, and ulcers. In this fresh, sweet-smelling salve, they soothe problem cuticles.

If you like the effects of the apricot oil, but you would rather use it in the form of a salve, you might prefer Apricot Oil-Lanolin Cuticle Salve. (See page 56 for the recipe.)

Castor Oil

Believe it or not, castor oil—a substance feared by generations of children—can benefit your cuticles and nails. Don't worry, you don't have to *drink* the castor oil to have beautiful nails! You just have to rub it in. This is one of my favorite treatments because it has a very smooth, unctuous quality, and yet isn't greasy. It also has a pleasant smell—one that might remind you of lipstick, as many lipsticks contain this oil.

To use this wonderful oil, just massage a dab into each nail and cuticle every day. Gently finish rubbing the oil in with a tissue. Your cuticles will be soft and supple, and your nails will look shiny and healthy all day. (For more information on castor oil, see Chapter 5.)

HEALING A HANGNAIL

Hangnails are unsightly, and a really bad one can tear right into the cuticle, causing pain and bleeding. So if a hangnail appears, it's wise to take steps to heal and treat it as quickly as possible. In earlier chapters, I've mentioned using white iodine for hangnails, but white iodine stings when applied to a big, bad, bleeding hangnail. So I've developed a strategy for healing the hangnail and drying it up almost completely within three days with a minimum of stinging and trauma.

As soon as possible after you notice the hangnail, wash your hands thoroughly with an antibacterial soap and warm water. This is one time when the use of an antibacterial soap makes sense, as a severe hangnail is a convenient port of entry for bacteria.

That evening, gently rub vitamin E oil from a capsule onto the hangnail. Vitamin E has been shown to speed the healing of fresh cuts and wounds, and is perfect for treating nasty new hangnails. By the next morning, you may be surprised to see how much better the hangnail is!

The *next* night, apply the white iodine to your hangnail. This will dry up and further disinfect the area. And at this point, it will sting only a bit.

On the third night, take a piece of grapefruit peel and rub the white pith over the hangnail. The vitamin C and other antioxidant compounds in the grapefruit oil will promote further healing. By this time, the hangnail will have practically vanished. Thank goodness!

You might also want to try applying tea tree oil to an inflamed hangnail. Although a powerful natural antiseptic, tea tree oil is mild enough to be used undiluted by a carrier oil on all but the most sensitive skin.

Whatever you do, don't bite the hangnail off! This sounds horrible, looks horrible, and *is* horrible. The entire cuticle area can become inflamed and sore. A nail clipper stashed in your purse or pocket can be used to nip off the ragged end of a hangnail so that it doesn't get worse during the day. (Just be sure to avoid cutting into the living tissue!) Then try to wash your hands as soon as possible and smooth some waxy lip balm over any raggedness on the cuticle.

Your nails probably look healthier now than they have in years. Chips and splits have been sent on their way, and your four-part regimen is sloughing away dead cuticle cells and strengthening your nails. Your cuticles are being moisturized, smoothed, and shaped. But perhaps your nails are already beginning to grow out. What to do? Read on, and you'll learn how to file your nails so that they are as graceful and flattering as they are healthy.

Chapter 4

Shaping Your Nails Beautifully

S o far we've concentrated on nail and cuticle health and grooming. Your cuticles should be looking much smoother and neater by now than they did a few weeks ago, and your nails should be stronger and glossier. Finally, it's time to think about nail length and shape.

As you have already discovered, my own preference is for short nails. Short, meticulously groomed nails can be refined, lovely, and *very* feminine. However, you may prefer your nails to be somewhat longer in length. Whatever length you choose, your nails will have to be filed to maintain that length *and* to maintain an attractive shape. Filing nails into a pretty shape is an art. Some of us can do it naturally. Others need to learn. That's what this chapter is about. In the following pages, you'll learn about the tools that will help you file your nails without compromising their health. You'll learn about choosing the best shape and length for your own nails. You'll be led step by step through the manicure process. And finally, once those new healthy nails are perfectly filed, you'll learn how to maintain their appearance even when splits and chips throw obstacles in your path.

CHOOSING THE BEST NAIL FILE

Before you begin to consider nail shape and length, you'll want to buy the best nail file for the job. Files are all fairly inexpensive, so you can experiment with a variety and see what works best on your nails. Keep in mind that the quality of your file will definitely affect the ease and accuracy of your filing. No matter how good your technique, a poor-quality file can lead to uneven, ragged results and weakened nails.

Files Used for Shaping

I feel that the best nail file you can use to shape your nails is a metal nail file coated with diamond or sapphire dust. Fine, hard abrasives, gem dusts will file your nails accurately and cleanly with a minimum of fraying even if your nails are soft.

Depending on your nails, though, you may find that other files also produce satisfactory results. A good-quality emery board is acceptable for nails of average or above-average hardness and strength. Just be sure to toss away these boards the instant they become worn. Also avoid buying inexpensive cardboard files, as they are usually too coarse and gritty to file your nails with gentle precision, and also tend to be unevenly coated with abrasive. "Micrograin" coatings, like gem-dust coatings, offer a fine abrasive surface. Cushioned nail files are also available, with a soft layer sandwiched between the two cardboard filing surfaces. Because these files "give" more as you work and are usually well made, they are a good choice for some fragile nails. You might also want to try cardboard nail files that contain "protein conditioners." When I first saw these, I regarded the conditioners as a silly gimmick. But these files do seem to file very smoothly.

You might have seen metal or plastic files coated with three different grades of abrasives. *Never* use the coarse grade—it's meant for filing tough artificial nails. Medium grit is okay for nails of average or above-average hardness, and fine grit works well for fragile nails. In fact, if you have fragile nails, you should almost always use the fine side of any file—even a sapphire- or diamond-coated file.

Files Used for Smoothing

One of two types of files can be used to smooth the edges of your nails once you have shaped them with a regular file. The first is an implement called a hindostone, a thick file made of a smooth, stonelike material. The second, which is sometimes referred to as a fine sander, is a small disk-shaped file made of cardboard that has been coated with a very fine abrasive. Either of these files will give your nails a beautifully smooth, finished look; choose whichever one you prefer.

Ridge Sanders

Finally, if your nails are heavily ridged, you might want to look into ridge sanders. Ridge sanders are heavy duty files used to sand down any ridges that run vertically from the cuticle to the nail tip. Heavy ridging seems to be a hereditary trait, although some nutritionists say it's a sign of poor nutrition. Whatever their cause, ridges are troublesome to some women. Ridge sanders literally sand down the surface of the nail, making it smoother and more even. However, in doing so, these sanders also make the nail thinner and, of course, weaker. So this option should be chosen only if the ridges are heavy, and should not be used more than once a month. Remember that some slight ridging is normal even in healthy nails.

A Final Word on Files

No matter how high in quality your nail file, keep in mind that no file lasts forever. A good gem-coated file can last for about six to eight months. A good-quality cardboard file might last for only one month. If you're ever unsure if your file is too worn for proper filing, simply run the pad of your index finger lightly down the file's surface. The abrasive should feel evenly distributed over the file. If you can feel the worn spots, it's time for a new file.

CHOOSING NAIL LENGTH AND SHAPE

How long should you let your nails grow? While you're initially repairing and strengthening your nails and cuticles, you'll want to keep your nails as short as possible—certainly no longer than fingertip length. But once your nails have become smoother and stronger, you might consider growing them a bit longer.

The nail length you select can depend on a variety of factors. The first consideration is the hardness of your nails. If you have fragile nails, it's best not to let them grow beyond the tips of your fingers. This will both stabilize the nail and present a graceful appearance, without impeding you in your daily activities. Women with stronger, harder nails can afford to grow their nails longer without being concerned about splitting and chipping as they perform their daily tasks.

Another consideration is your job and your hobbies. My hobbies include gardening, cooking, and painting in oils—the last of which couldn't be worse for nail health. So I usually keep my nails no more than fingertip length. This is especially important in the winter, when harsh weather and drying indoor heating present real problems for fragile nails like mine. If your hobbies or your job is hard on nails, a shorter length will allow you to consistently maintain a neat and healthy appearance.

You'll also want to consider the overall look of your hands and nails. The more fine-boned your hands are, the shorter your nails can be without looking stubby. The squarer and larger-boned your hands are, the longer you might want to grow your nails. In addition, longer nail beds give even closely trimmed nails the appearance of length and grace. If your nail beds are shorter, a longer length might be more flattering.

Finally, you'll want to decide on nail shape. There are several basic nail shapes from which you can choose. (See Figure 4.1.)

For the first shape, you create a curve that echoes the curve of your nail bed. This is particularly good for soft nails, as it will keep your nails as strong as possible.

For the second shape, you file the nail into a more pronounced oval shape. A graceful look, this does require a somewhat stronger nail.

"Squaring" the nails—the third approach—is a more sporty look. On some hands, it looks very attractive and finished. And like the first nail shaped discussed, this one is an excellent choice for fragile nails.

Yet a fourth approach is to shape the nail so that the curve mirrors the curve of the cuticle. While this is a balanced, harmonious look, quite frankly, it is for advanced filers—not for the filing-impaired.

When choosing a shape for your nail, you might want to glance through a fashion magazine and find a model with

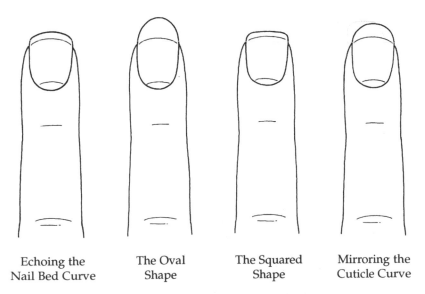

| Echoing the
Nail Bed Curve | The Oval
Shape | The Squared
Shape | Mirroring the
Cuticle Curve |

Figure 4.1 The Four Basic Nail Shapes

A Brief History of Nail Fashion

Throughout history, nails have been used as fashion statements and status symbols. It is both fascinating and fun to see how nail length, shape, and color have changed over the centuries, reflecting changing cultures and values, and telling us a great deal about how we view ourselves.

Ancient Egyptians were very nail conscious, a fact testified to by the elaborate sets of solid gold manicure implements found in Egyptian tombs. Both in the name of fashion and to repel evil spirits, Cleopatra used henna to tint her nails, her fingertips, and even the palms of her hands!

The Longest Fingernails in History Award goes to the upper class Chinese of the seventeenth century. Women and men alike grew five-inch-long fingernails designed to proclaim, "I live a life of leisure." Elaborate jeweled gold or bamboo splints prevented these curving claws from breaking, and it's fortunate that the invention of the telephone lay far in the future.

The custom of having long nails spread over much of the Far East, and centuries later, the Dragon Lady appeared as a character in the World War II-era comic strip Terry and the Pirates. Even now, we refer to "Dragon Lady talons" when describing long red fingernails.

Courtiers at Versailles in seventeenth-century France grew the little-finger nail of only *one* hand long. Why? So that they could scratch on a door instead of knocking—an act that was considered unspeakably gauche. Etiquette prescribed that the courtier scratch the door softly and delicately.

During the nineteenth century, a nail shape called the "filbert" was all the rage. This was an oval shape with a slightly more pointed tip than we are accustomed to now. Upper class English women in the early nineteenth century used a subtle rose nail powder to color their nails, but even that was too much for Queen Victoria, who let it be known that she was not amused. Nail powder and other cosmetics disappeared from the scene during her mid- to late-nineteenth century reign—a reign that seemed interminable to fashionable women.

World War I led to many social changes, including revolutions in women's dress and grooming. Nail enamels arrived on the fashion scene in the early twenties, having been developed from lacquers originally formulated as automotive paint. Brightly colored nails quickly developed working class connotations, and upper class women were warned against such garishness. But influential fashion designer Coco Chanel loved red fingernails, and once Jean Harlow simmered on the silver screen as an icon of glamour with long red nails, white satin gowns, and platinum blond hair, her signature nails reigned supreme. It was during this time that artificial nails were first developed. Made out of crude plastics, they enabled Hollywood stars to create the illusion of glamour on camera.

Remember Twiggy? Her frosted lipstick and nails revolutionized fashion first in swinging London, and later the world over. Long red nails, suddenly old hat, could be heard toppling all over the world. Then, in America, the Woodstock generation clipped off—or perhaps bit off—their fingernails and threw away their nail polish. The natural look was in.

By the early seventies, Raquel Welch and Barbra Streisand's long, beige, and obviously false nails had their influence. The "squared" nail shape became popular, a supposedly sporty look—although with nails easily a half an inch long, it was difficult to imagine a sport that might be played without doing great damage to both the nails and the players.

Life got serious in the eighties, and along with ties and navy suits, aspiring career women were supposed to have serious nails, subdued in color and modest in length. Such sober moderation could last only so long, though, and the early nineties saw the return of red nails— although this time, they were short.

Now we live in a time of choice, but whether you wear your nails long or short, brightly colored or softly natural, you want them to be strong, pliable, and healthy. Your Beautiful Hands and Nails Regimen will help you do just that, and will enable your hands to look their best regardless of the current fashions.

nails that you find pretty. Then use that picture as your shaping guide. Just be sure that the model you choose has hands and nails somewhat similar to your own. If not, your attempts may be frustrating.

Whatever shape you choose, be aware that getting the perfect shape for each nail may take considerably more than one or two sessions with the nail file. This is because each nail has its own unique shape. Additional nail brushing, too, might be needed to smooth and even out the curve of the nail beds.

Fortunately, nails grow quickly, so you will have ample opportunity to try different nail shapes and to perfect the shape that you eventually choose.

FILING YOUR NAILS

Before you begin to shape your nails, look at the ends of your nail beds. If you have been regularly brushing under your nails, they should be smooth and evenly rounded. If they aren't smooth and even, gently use an orange stick under the nail tip to smooth any unevenness. By the way, this is the only use I can think of for an orange stick, as poking at your cuticles with one of these implements can result in white spots and "mysterious" horizontal ridges in the nail. Even if the tip of the orange stick is padded with cotton, the potential for injury is there.

I've mentioned that some of us have a natural talent for shaping pretty nails. Those of use who aren't "naturals" may have haphazardly sawed away at our nails, ending up with some too short, some lopsided, or some roughened. A week later, we're reaching for nail clippers to clip off a jagged edge. But we never seem to achieve beautifully shaped nails.

Fortunately, by using a step-by-step approach, you can make your nails symmetrical, harmonious, and very flattering. Below, you will find a simple-to-follow guide to filing your nails into the easiest-to-create, most basic shape—a curve that echoes the shape of the nail bed. Following this, you will find directions for modifying these basic steps to create the other shapes we've discussed.

Basic Filing—Echoing the Nail Bed Curve

1. Begin filing the tip of the nail by holding the file parallel to the curve of the nail bed. Tilt the file slightly back (see Figure 4.2) so that you slightly bevel the edges of the nail. This will minimize fraying of the nail fibers. Filing gently in one direction, file the nail to the desired length.

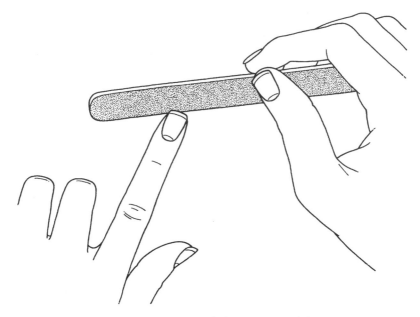

Figure 4.2 Angling the Nail File

As you file your nails, tilt the file back slightly—
about 30 degrees—to bevel the nail edge.

2. Now file one side of the nail roughly parallel to the side curve of the fingertip. Do the same on the other side of the nail. Do not curve in the entire side of the nail. Instead, after the nail emerges from the finger, allow it to grow out straight for a short distance—about a sixteenth of an inch—for added strength. Just a few strokes will suffice when filing the delicate sides.

3. Now that you have "roughed out" the nail shape, you should have four points on the nail. (See Figure 4.3.) The lowest two points are found where the lowest part of the side of the nail, which you have allowed to grow straight, meets the portion that has been slightly curved. The upper two points are found where the curved sides meet the slightly rounded top of the nail. File the points down to create a continuous curve.

4. At this point, you may notice some little tags of nail that

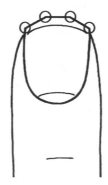

Figure 4.3 The Four File Points

After you rough out the shape of your nail, you should have four
file points. Smooth these points down to create a smooth curve.

extend beyond the nail edge. These are some of the nail fiber
layers that didn't get completely filed off. Use either a very
fine-grit circular file or a hindostone to smooth the edges,
eliminating any fraying.

5. Gently run the tip of each nail over a cake of white beeswax.
This will seal the fibers of the nail together and help to waterproof the nail, as well. Do not omit this step, as it is very effective in preventing splitting. As a final check, brush your nails
over an old pair of pantyhose. As you probably know, pantyhose are great nail-roughness detectors! If you detect a tiny burr
or nick, use your smoothing file—the circular file or hindostone—to eliminate the remaining roughness. Now you're done!

Creating an Oval Shape

Instead of beginning with your file parallel to the nail bed, first
file the two sides of the nail tip at a slight angle. As described in
the basic instructions above, you'll want to avoid curving in the
entire side of the nail. Instead, allow the nail to grow out
straight for a short distance for added strength. Then hold the
file parallel to the nail bed at the very tip of the nail, and file

Tips for Successfully Shaping Your Nails

This chapter presents step-by-step instructions for creating nails that are attractively and symmetrically shaped. In addition to these instructions, a few tricks of the trade will help you achieve the most pleasing, professional results the next time you give yourself a manicure.

❑ Before you begin the shaping process, visualize the desired nail shape. This mental image can serve as a useful guide, helping you create the shape you want.

❑ File your nails under strong, direct light so that you can clearly see what you're doing. If desired, occasionally use a hand-held magnifying glass to check the smoothness of your filing. Even tiny, almost invisible nicks can sometimes turn into big snags.

❑ Make sure that your file is of good quality and in good condition. If your file seems worn, discard it, and use a fresh one. (For more about files, see page 62.)

❑ As you file, tilt the file slightly under your nail, rather than holding it straight. This can help prevent fraying, resulting in a cleaner edge.

❑ File gently and lightly, allowing the abrasives to work for you. Avoid pressing hard with the file, as this can lead to fraying.

❑ Avoid filing down the nail where it emerges from the skin, as this can result in splits at the side of the nail. Instead, allow the nail to grow straight for about a sixteenth of an inch (see the figure below), and *then* begin creating the curve you desire. This will make your nail stronger, helping to prevent splits and breaks.

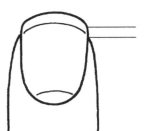

After the nail emerges from the finger, allow it to grow straight for $1/16$ of an inch before you begin filing it into a curve. This will give it added strength.

❏ Rather than using a sawing motion as you file, gently file each portion of the nail in one direction only. This doesn't mean that, for instance, you should file from left to right on each nail. Rather, file first from the left side to the center, and then from the right side to the center. This will create less wear on the nail edge and prevent fraying.

❏ Although it may be tempting to omit the last two steps of the filing process—namely, smoothing the nails and running them across beeswax—it is vital to include these steps in every filing session. By spending a few extra moments smoothing and sealing your nail tips, you can help prevent snags and breaks in the days to come.

smoothly. This will result in a rough oval—again, a shape accented by four points. File any points down to form a smooth curve, and finish the nail with smoothing files and beeswax as described in the basic directions.

Creating a Squared Shape

Begin by following the instructions for creating an oval nail. Then gently file off just the curving *tip* of the nail to achieve a flat, straight nail tip. You might want to flatten off the curve just slightly so that the nail is squared only slightly, or you might prefer to file off more of the curve for a more pronounced squaring. Allow your own taste to be your guide. Finally, finish the nail with smoothing files and beeswax as described in the basic directions.

Mirroring the Curve of the Cuticle

Begin by looking carefully at the shape of the cuticle of the nail you are shaping. In most cases, the cuticle forms a rounded oval. Follow the instructions for creating an oval nail, keeping the exact shape of the cuticle in mind. I find it helpful to visualize the completed nail, and to use that image as a guide during the shaping process. Then finish the nail with the smoothing file and beeswax according to the basic instructions.

BEING A FREQUENT FILER

When you're finished filing your nails, they should, ideally, be harmonious in shape and length. But, as I've said before, nails grow fast! Before you know it, the most rapidly growing nails such as those of your little fingers can outstrip the others in size, and your hands can become a hodgepodge of overgrown nails that will need a lengthy filing session to restore their pleasing appearance.

The solution? Be a frequent filer. By lightly filing your nails on a frequent basis, you can avoid finding yourself with a mismatched assortment of lengths and shapes. Light, frequent filing is also easier on nails than occasional heavy filing. This doesn't mean that you have to have a long filing session every day. But, especially during the spring and summer months when nail growth speeds up, you should lightly file your nails for just a few moments every few days—perhaps while watching TV or just before going to bed.

Eventually, of course, your nails may "get away from you," and you will again find yourself with a motley collection. When this happens, file them all to the length of the *shortest* nail, clipping the longest ones with nail clippers if they've become too long to file. There's no reason to try to preserve the longest nails just because they're long. Look at your hand as a single entity, and keep all your nails the same general length and shape. The result will be a harmonious and immaculate appearance.

PREVENTING AND CARING
FOR SPLITS AND CHIPS

So now you have perfectly filed nails—or are well on your way to learning to file them perfectly. Great! And I bet your ooking better and better with each passing day. But you do if you glance down at your nails, and, horrors, a nail is chipping or splitting? Will you quickly put on a pair of white gloves? Hide your hands under the table? Fortunately, such drastic means are not necessary—not if you have a jar of Beeswax Nail Spackle on hand! But before we look at nail repair, let's see what you can do to help prevent chips and splits from occurring in the first place.

Preventing Nail Damage

To avoid major nail breaks, try to use your nails as carefully as possible. For instance, avoid using them as screwdrivers, scrapers, or any other tools. Use the proper tools, instead. And in the kitchen, be sure to exercise great care when using hand graters, knives, and other implements that can grate or slice off a portion of your nail.

When appropriate, wear gloves to protect your hands from chemicals and water. For instance, if you refinish furniture with paint remover, buy and *use* the gloves made especially for that purpose. Similarly, when doing dishes, try to wear rubber dishwashing gloves. If these gloves seem too clumsy, keep a small jar of petroleum jelly or Calendula Cuticle Salve (page 57) by the sink, and apply a film of the product to your nails and hands before beginning your task. This will prevent the splitting and fraying that can occur when nails soak up hot, soapy dishwater.

You may notice that splits and breaks always occur in the same place on the same nails. For instance, I have two areas prone to splitting on the right half of both thumbnails. If you observe problem areas like this on your own nails, practice preventive nail care by keeping any rough edges in these areas smoothly filed, and by applying your nail protector to the breakage-prone spots. For further preventive care, apply a little petroleum jelly or another nail nourisher to the *underside* of the nail tip. This is particularly important if you keep your nails longer than fingertip length. The nail tips—the oldest, driest part of the nail—tend to be vulnerable to splitting, and can use that added protection.

Treating Nail Damage

Despite your best efforts, your fragile nails may occasionally chip and split. If they are already fairly short and you don't want to make them any shorter, you may be looking longingly at a bottle of nail hardener now. But wait! Help is on the way.

Beeswax, which we've mentioned in previous chapters, is a wonderful substance—natural, waterproof, and quite happily produced by honeybees. Unfortunately, in its pure form, beeswax is quite hard and crumbles if stroked across the nail. But if you melt the beeswax with a small amount of jojoba oil and then allow it to reharden, a wonderful thing occurs. You create Beeswax Nail Spackle—a salve that is very firm, yet easy to spread over the nail, and that can act as both nail protection and a sort of glue. Better yet, Beeswax Nail Spackle is easy to make at home using the recipe on page 76.

Once you've made your own jar of Beeswax Nail Spackle, you'll find it an invaluable nail care aid. When you see a hangnail in the making, scrape off some of the salve with the tip of your index fingernail and spread it over the cuticle. Do the same for a nail that is beginning to chip. If a small split occurs, again, apply a coating of the salve to the area, "gluing" the edges together. Eventually, as the nail grows longer, you'll be able to file the break away.

Although, as the name implies, Beeswax Nail Spackle was designed chiefly to spackle problem areas, it also works well as a preventive measure. If certain nails are prone to cracks—and especially if you're involved in chores of a nail-threatening nature—spread the salve thickly on the nail and cuticle. You may hesitate to use this much, but the salve is almost invisible. The only drawback might be that it can't be buffed to a high shine. However, I find its soft sheen attractive.

Making Beeswax Nail Spackle

Of all the nail-care products that you can make using the recipes in this book, Beeswax Nail Spackle is perhaps the most unique. Although made entirely of natural ingredients, it actually has the ability to *mend* small chips and splits, preserving the appearance of your nails until any problem area grows out. Plus it can be used to protect your nails from water and damaging chemicals.

Fortunately, Beeswax Nail Spackle is a snap to make. Just follow the simple directions below.

Beeswax Nail Spackle

Yield: 1 tablespoon

¼ ounce white beeswax, chipped*
½ teaspoon jojoba oil

*Cut a 1-ounce cylinder or cube of beeswax into four equal parts to get ¼ ounce.

1. Place both ingredients in a heatproof cup or bowl. (If desired, use the container you will store the mixture in, as long as it's heatproof.) Then place the container in a small saucepan, and pour water into the pan until it's about halfway up the side of the container.

2. Place the saucepan over low heat, bring the water to a simmer, and heat until the beeswax melts completely, occasionally stirring with the tip of a knife. Be sure not to leave the pan unattended.

3. Allow the mixture to cool to room temperature, and check the consistency. If it's too thick to spread, add a bit more oil and remelt it. When cool, cover and store at room temperature, using as desired.

After you've used your jar of Beeswax Nail Spackle for a time, you might want to create your own special spackle formula. Beeswax has to be the main ingredient, of course, but you can replace the jojoba oil with another oil, such as apricot kernel oil. You can also add a few drops of vitamin E oil, or even a drop of an essential oil such as violet or patchouli.

Now your nails are clean, healthy, and beautifully shaped. And you've gotten them this way without the use of caustic exfoliators or artificial hardeners and polishes. But there may be times when you want to showcase your beautiful hands by adding just a touch of shine and color. The next chapter will show you how to do just that—naturally, of course!

Chapter 5

Nail Color and Shine

At this point, if you've been following your four-part regimen for two or three weeks, your nails should be much improved and, for all intents and purposes, invisible. What do I mean by *invisible*? Invisible nails are neat, smooth, and clean, and neither add to nor detract from your appearance. Don't sneer at invisible nails. For some professions, they're exactly what you want. Doctors, nurses, chefs, dentists, even hairstylists are probably best sporting invisible nails. In fact, in any profession in which you physically touch people or prepare food, plain, immaculate nails are attractive and confidence inspiring.

As tidy and professional-looking as invisible nails can be, most of us at least sometimes want nails with a bit more pizzazz. In this chapter, we'll look at gentle ways to shine, color, and otherwise enhance the appearance of your nails using only natural substances.

WHITENING YOUR NAILS

No matter how wonderfully strong, healthy, and well-shaped your nails are, if they are yellowed, they will not be attractive.

Why might nails turn yellow? A number of habits, including smoking, can cause marked nail yellowing. Even the simple passage of time causes a gradual, imperceptible yellowing. Fortunately, there are simple ways to make your nails look whiter and cleaner. The first, a bleach made with hydrogen peroxide, will actually lift some of the stain out of your nails. The second, a nail-whitening pencil, will give just the tips of your nails a whiter appearance.

Bleaching Your Nails

If you would like to have very clean-looking nails, try bleaching them gently with a mixture of hydrogen peroxide and baking soda. Simply place 1 tablespoon of 3-percent hydrogen peroxide and 2 ½ tablespoons of baking soda in a small non-metal bowl, and mix the ingredients into a paste. Then use a cotton swab to press some of the mixture firmly under the tip of each nail as well as over the top of the nail, covering all the nails on one hand. Allow the mixture to remain in place for two to three minutes, no longer. Then rinse the bleach off with warm water. If any particles of the mixture remain after rinsing, brush under the nails with your natural bristle nail brush. Repeat with the other hand. Finish by massaging a dab of petroleum jelly into each nail. Use this treatment no more than every six to eight weeks.

Like other substances that have a bleaching effect—including lemon juice and buttermilk—hydrogen peroxide has the potential to irritate skin and nails if left in contact with them for too long a time. For this reason, it is important not to exceed the two- to three-minute treatment time. If you want to use this treatment more frequently than the suggested six to eight weeks, evaluate your nails carefully after use for signs of splitting and drying. And, of course, be sure to use nothing stronger than the 3-percent solution of hydrogen peroxide. Hydrogen peroxide has long been used as a mild skin antiseptic, and will not harm your skin and nails as long as you follow these guidelines.

Using a Nail-Whitening Pencil

If you prefer not to use bleach on your nails, or if you want a brighter, more opaque look, you might like the effects of a commercial nail-whitening pencil. When you buy the pencil, be sure to buy a pencil sharpener, as for good results, the pencil tip must be kept sharp. To use the pencil, place the sharpened tip under the nail tip. Be sure to hold the tip against the *nail*, not the finger. For best results, rest your hand on a tabletop to steady it as you whiten your nails. Then run the pencil along the underside of the nail tip, moving it from one side of the nail to the other. (See Figure 5.1.) As necessary, stop to resharpen the pencil every few nails, as this process is easiest when the pencil has a good point.

Even if you don't think that your nails need whitening, you might want to try either nail bleaching or a nail-whitening pencil. White nail tips really do present a sharper, more finished appearance. You will love the results!

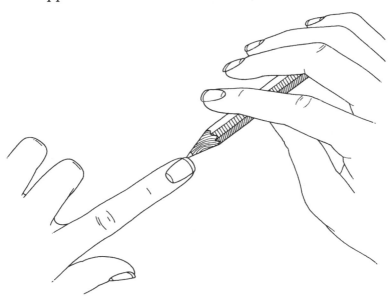

Figure 5.1 Using a Nail-Whitening Pencil

Run the nail-whitening pencil along the underside
of the nail tip, moving it from one side to the other.

SHINING YOUR NAILS

By using a natural method to add shine to your nails, you will subtly showcase their beauty without making them look artificial. No garish color. Just a healthy sheen.

There are two different ways to make your nails shine. The first is to buff your nails. The second is to apply an oil that adds smoothness and gloss.

Buffing Your Nails

Nail buffing is the old-fashioned way to polish and shine nails. Of course, the results are not as long-lasting as nail polish, but, on the other hand, a buffed shine doesn't chip, never requires the use of drying nail polish removers, and lends your nails a subtle, lovely sheen. When beeswax is used, the shine from nail buffing can last for three or four days, depending on how often you immerse your hands in water. In addition, daily gentle buffing increases circulation to the nails, possibly stimulating growth. And if that isn't reason enough to use this old-time technique, buffing adds a thin, hard layer to your nails, helping to strengthen them.

You can buff your nails with one of two types of polish: nail buffing cream and beeswax.

Nail buffing creams can be found at most drugstores and beauty supply stores. Buffing cream contains finely ground abrasives that polish the nail as you would polish a jewel. The cream can be used either with a special nail buffer—also available at drug and beauty stores—or with a small piece of chamois, which you can find at any hardware store.

To buff your nails with buffing cream, apply a tiny dab of buffing cream to the nail and buff in only one direction using either a buffer or a chamois. Polishing your nails in one direction only will prevent you from buffing too quickly, causing the nail to "burn"—to feel uncomfortably warm. For an especially hard and glossy shine, apply two thin coats of buffing cream, buffing thoroughly after each coat. Your nails will have a beautiful sheen.

Beeswax will give your nails a harder, longer-lasting shine than you can get with a nail buffing cream. To use it, simply rub a piece of white beeswax over the nail, and buff as directed above. Be aware that you can't use Beeswax Nail Spackle for this purpose—only pure beeswax.

Shining Your Nails With Myrrh Oil

In Chapter 3, you learned how certain aromatherapy oils can help to heal and soften dry, roughened cuticles. One of these fragrant oils—myrrh oil—can also lend your nails a subtle sheen, added hardness, and even a delightfully exotic scent!

Myrrh oil is extracted from the resin of a Middle Eastern shrub called *Balsamodenron myrrha*. One of the original perfumes ever used—it's mentioned in writings that date back 2,700 years!—myrrh oil has a subtle, slightly musky scent, with undertones of cedar and spice. An infection fighter and immune booster, myrrh has also long been valued for its medicinal properties. And while many essential oils can be irritating to your skin, myrrh oil is gentle enough to be used undiluted.

Like other essential oils, myrrh oil can be purchased wherever aromatherapy oils are sold. Or you can order it by mail. (See the Resource List on page 133.) I recommend buying only an eighth of an ounce to begin with, as this relatively thin oil lasts for a long time.

To use myrrh oil as a nail shiner, place a tiny drop on each nail, and rub it in. If desired, you can intensify the shine by buffing with a nail buffer or a chamois. Your nails will both gleam *and* smell wonderful!

By the way, you might be interested to learn that there is a time-honored tradition of using myrrh on fingertips. A love poem in the Song of Solomon contains these lines:

I rose to open to my beloved,
    and my hands dripped with myrrh,
my fingers with liquid myrrh . . .

Shining Your Nails With Castor Oil

In Chapter 3, I discussed how castor oil can help soothe and moisturize dry, hard cuticles. Well, this wonderful oil will also add gloss to your nails! Simply place a tiny dab on each nail, and gently rub in for smooth, shiny nails *and* healthy cuticles.

If you like what castor oil does for your nails, you might want to concoct your own custom nail-glossing mixture. My favorite is a mixture of equal parts of castor oil and jojoba oil, plus the contents of a vitamin E capsule and a vitamin A capsule. You might also want to add a few drops of tea tree oil. Just don't get too enthusiastic and mix up too much, as a little goes a long, long way. Try using a few teaspoons of each oil, and store your formula in a labelled empty aspirin bottle. Shiny nails couldn't be easier!

COLORING YOUR NAILS NATURALLY

You may be surprised to learn that you can actually color your nails without using commercial nail products or other artificial substances. Three types of coloring agents are available. The first, henna, is a permanent dye. Alkanet powder, the second option, will tint your nails for several days. Finally, there's lip pencils, which will add color for up to two days.

Using Henna

It takes courage to use henna tint on your nails for the first time. After all, henna is a dye, not a coating, and cannot be removed. But I urge the adventurous, curious, and fearless among you to take the plunge. You may love the pale peach hue it gives to your nails.

Using Henna As a Natural Nail Hardener

Earlier in the chapter, I explained how you can use red henna to naturally tint your nails a subtle, lovely peach color. But henna has other uses, as well. When used in its colorless form, henna, which contains a resinous substance, can actually strengthen your nails, helping to prevent splits, chips, and tears.

Like red henna, neutral henna may be found in health foods stores, usually packaged as a hair conditioner. Before using this product, take the allergy test described on page 86. Then proceed as follows:

1. Scrub your nails using a mild liquid castile soap. For best results, you want your nails to be oil-, wax-, and perspiration-free. Then dry your hands and nails carefully.

2. Place 1 tablespoon of neutral henna and 1½ tablespoons of warm water in a glass bowl, and stir with a spoon until well mixed. The result will look something like mud.

3. Using a small round-tipped knife, take a dab of the henna and apply it to an entire nail, including the filed edges. This is a bit like applying a tiny mud pack to each nail. You may wish to use a cotton swab to press the henna mixture onto the nails. Don't worry about covering your cuticles, as neutral henna can't stain them. Repeat on all of the remaining nails. (Unlike red henna, neutral henna can be applied to all nails at once.)

4. Allow the henna pack to remain on the nails for three to five minutes. Then rinse the nails well with warm water, using a nail brush if desired to remove all of the henna particles.

5. Dry your hands well, and buff with a nail buffer or chamois to shine up the resin coating on the nail. To prevent a buildup of resin, use no more than once a month.

Henna is prepared from the dried, ground leaves of the *Lawsonia inermis,* a Middle Eastern shrub. For thousands of years, it has been used both as a cosmetic dye and as a dye for fabrics and leather. Henna dye can be found in the cosmetic section of your local health foods store, where it is sold as a hair dye. Look for packages labelled "henna" or "red henna." Neutral henna, which will *not* add color to your nails, is labelled as such on the package. (To learn how to use neutral henna as a nail strengthener, see the inset on page 85.)

If you have never used henna before, and if you are prone to allergies, you might want to try this product on a toenail before using it on your fingers. Apply it for several minutes, rinse it off, and wait twenty-four hours to check for a reaction. In fact, if you're at all hesitant about using henna on your fingernails, try it on your toenails first. This is a great way to see if you like the effect! If you do, just follow these easy directions:

1. First scrub your nails using a mild liquid castile soap. You want your nails to be oil-, wax-, and perspiration-free, or else the tint may be mottled. Then dry your hands and nails carefully.

2. Place 1 tablespoon of henna and 1½ tablespoons of warm water in a glass bowl—not a metal bowl or a bowl that can be stained by the dye—and stir with a spoon until well mixed. The result will look something like mud. Set aside.

3. Using a cotton swab, cover your cuticles with a light film of petroleum jelly. This will help prevent them from being stained by the henna.

4. Using a small round-tipped knife, take a dab of the henna and apply it to the entire nail. Include the filed edge, but avoid the cuticles. This is a bit like applying a tiny mud pack to each nail. You may wish to use a cotton swab to press the henna mixture onto the nails. Repeat on only one other nail. (For even results, it's best to dye only two nails at a time.)

5. Allow the henna pack to remain on the nails for three to five minutes. Then rinse the nails well with warm water, using a nail brush if desired to remove all of the henna particles. Repeat with two more nails at a time until all of your nails are dyed.

6. When all of your nails have been tinted, dry your hands well and buff with a nail buffer or chamois. Buffing shines up the resin coating on the nail.

The method detailed above will give your nails a barely perceptible tint. If you like the effect but want a more pronounced result, the next time, try leaving the henna pack on for another minute or two.

If you feel "all thumbs" when applying henna, try inviting a friend over and tinting each other's nails. Moroccan women have been doing this for centuries, and turn the occasion into a party. In fact, women have used henna to dye their entire fingertips and even the soles of their feet. Be the first on your block!

Using Alkanet Powder

Alkanet is an herb that grows wild in southern Europe. Its root contains a dye that is chemically similar to henna. Unlike henna, though, alkanet will lend your nails a delicate rosy hue, rather than a peach color.

As you might have guessed, alkanet powder is probably not available at your local health foods store or drugstore. However, if you have a local herb store, it may carry alkanet. This product can also be purchased from mail order companies that specialize in herbs. (See the Resource List on page 133.) Then tint your nails by following these simple directions.

1. First, scrub your nails using a mild liquid castile soap. You want your nails to be oil-, wax-, and perspiration-free, or else the tint may be mottled. Then dry your hands and nails completely.

2. Place a teaspoon of alkanet powder and a teaspoon of 70-percent isopropyl rubbing alcohol in a small glass dish, and stir to form a smooth paste. Set aside.

3. Using a cotton swab, cover your cuticles with a light film of petroleum jelly. This will help prevent them from being stained.

4. Using a clean cotton swab, apply the alkanet mixture to the fingers of one hand. Include the filed edge, but avoid the cuti-

cles. Do not allow the dye to remain on your nails. Instead, when you've finished applying the alkanet paste to the nails of one hand, rinse it off under running water, using a nail brush and some castile soap to remove any excess paste. Repeat with the nails of the other hand. When all of your nails have been tinted, dry your hands well.

If you've followed the above instructions, your nails should have a delicate rose tint. If you would prefer a darker color, leave the alkanet on a bit longer—as long as one to two minutes. If your nails turn a bit too dark, or if you get some of the dye on a cuticle, don't worry. Unlike henna, alkanet wears off in a few days.

Using Lip Pencils

A simple and fun way to color your nails is to use lip pencils. These pencils are soft enough in texture to allow you to spread the color over your nails, but hard enough to remain on your nails without smearing. The effect of lip pencils is very subtle. Your nails will look incredibly healthy and rosy—natural, but somehow a bit better than natural. And, of course, you'll find a wide range of colors available, so that according to your mood, you can opt for anything from light pink to deep rose and sienna.

To use lip pencils on your nails, just lightly dot the nail with the pencil or draw a squiggle. Then gently massage the color evenly over the nail, right up to the cuticle. You might be tempted to use a buffer to add shine, but I've found that this buffs most of the color away. Instead, place a tiny dot of petroleum jelly, vitamin E oil, or myrrh oil on the colored nail, and gently massage it in. This will seal in the color and give it depth and shine.

Of the three methods of coloring your nails, this, of course, is the shortest lasting. If you protect your hands from strong soaps and detergents, though, the lip-penciled tint can last for about two days, gradually wearing away. This makes it perfect for a special occasion when you want your nails to look really fabulous. Then, when it's over, it's easy to remove any residue, if desired. Simply use your mild soap and a nail brush.

I hope I've inspired you to go beyond invisible nails—especially when it's so easy to have nails that are rosy, with a soft, healthy sheen. Beautiful!

Chapter 6

Protecting and Treating Your Hands

Far and few, far and few,
Are the lands where the Jumblies live;
Their heads are green, and their hands are blue,
And they went to sea in a sieve.

– Edward Lear, 1871

While most of us don't have the unusual hand problems of the Jumblies, many of us do have hands that are dry, rough, and perhaps reddened by countless hours of washing dishes, gardening, or other chores and pastimes, as well as by exposure to blazing sun and chilling cold. Many of us are also plagued by age spots—those ugly brown spots that appear on the backs of your hands. Fortunately, there is much you can do to prevent time, the elements, and the million and one tasks you perform from taking their toll on your appearance. And if your hands have already been marked by wear and by the passing years, there is much you can do to soothe, soften, and heal damaged skin, and even to gradually fade any age spots.

PREVENTIVE CARE FOR HANDS

If you have read the preceding chapters on nails, you may have already realized that it is far easier to prevent damage than it is to remedy it once it occurs. This is particularly true of hand care. Yes, dry, cracked skin can be moisturized, and age spots can be encouraged to fade. But it is so much easier to safeguard your hands in the first place than it is to reverse the ravages of time and abuse. Best of all, it is a relatively simple matter to provide your hands with the protection they need and deserve.

Gathering a Glove Wardrobe

One of the best ways you can protect the delicate skin on your hands is to gather a wardrobe of gloves. If you live in a temperate climate, you probably already own heavy gloves for those blustery winter months. But your hands will also benefit from protection on chilly spring and autumn days, so pamper them by buying a pair or two of lighter-weight gloves, as well. And on those days when frigid winds blow, wear the warmest gloves you can find. If your hands suffer from the cold even when wearing gloves, try thermal gloves that contain cotton. The cotton helps wick moisture from the skin. If you don't care for the utilitarian appearance of thermal gloves, try wearing them inside a pretty pair of mittens.

Exposure to detergents—as well as to cleaning solutions used to wash floors, counters, and the like—is one of the most common causes of dry, sore, chapped hands. The solution? Wear rubber gloves to protect your hands from hot water and detergents. If these gloves seem too cumbersome, buy latex gloves at your local drugstore. Thinner than rubber dishwashing gloves, these gloves give you greater flexibility and a better sense of "feel." Unfortunately, they are not as durable as rubber gloves, so that you'll want to buy several pairs at a time.

Due to the dehydrating effects of soil, gardening can also

take its toll, resulting in cracked skin, embedded dirt, and, of course, chipped nails. So if you love to garden—or even if you only run out a couple of times a year to plant flowers or to pull up a few weeds—it makes sense to invest in a pair or two of good gardening gloves. Use only gloves that are in good shape, tossing out any with holes. For further protection, before donning your gloves, rub a dab of petroleum jelly into each hand, especially on any calluses on the fingertips where dirt can become embedded. Then rub your nail tips lightly over a bar of soap to prevent any dirt that sifts through the gloves from getting under the nails. After your gardening session is over, scrub under your nails with a nail brush to remove the soap and any soil, as well.

If you're a gardening enthusiast, you know that certain delicate procedures such as thinning seedlings are difficult to perform using full gloves. Instead of doing them bare-handed, though, cut the fingertips off an old pair of gardening gloves, and wear them for any task that requires a bit more dexterity. They will not protect your nails and fingertips, but they will shield the backs of your hands from sun exposure.

Of course, many other tasks can also harm your hands—and your nails, too. If you color your own hair, be sure to wear the plastic gloves usually provided in the product package. They will prevent your hands from being stained by the dye. Similarly, be sure to use the proper gloves when refinishing furniture, painting walls, or doing any other work on your home or furniture.

Protecting Your Hands in Cold Weather

I've already mentioned that even on cool days, your hands can benefit from the use of gloves. The rule of thumb is: If it's cold enough to wear a jacket, it's cold enough to put those gloves on! Certainly, in the dead of winter, you'll want to keep your gloves on *every* time you leave the house.

Many of us find that our hands are cold even when we're *in* the house. If this is a problem for you, and if raising the thermostat is not an option, try wearing gloves without fingertips! Sometimes available in department stores—although they're more popular some years than others—these gloves will allow you to perform your usual tasks around the house or office. If you can't find these gloves in the stores, simply buy a pair of pretty but subdued-looking gardening gloves, and cut off the last inch or so of the fingers. Worn back in the nineteenth century, these mitts not only protect your hands from the cold, but help keep the rest of you toasty.

In Chapter 7, I will discuss the importance of exercise for the health of both hands and nails. During the cold weather, the increased circulation that exercise promotes will help pump the warmed blood to your hands and feet. Regular exercise will lend your hands a healthy glow, too.

If, despite a diligent use of gloves, you find that your hands are dry and chapped, a variety of treatments can be used to soothe and heal them. Especially effective is the Intensive Moisturizing Treatment (see page 101).

Protecting Your Hands in Warm Weather

If you're following the four-part regimen described in Chapter 2, your hands are always afforded some protection by the sunscreen in your hand cream. Although it is important to use a sunscreen-enriched hand cream even during the winter months—the sun's damaging rays reach your skin even on the coldest, most overcast days!—it is, of course, particularly important to do so during the summer, when the sun's rays are most direct and you're most likely to spend time outdoors. Remember that excess sun exposure is the number-one cause of rough, weather-beaten, age spot-marred hands. The glow of good health from suntanning is temporary, but the damage caused by sun exposure—especially the changes in skin texture—can be difficult to reverse.

It is also important to keep in mind that no sunscreen can

protect you *completely* from the damaging rays of the sun—especially if you spend long periods of time outdoors. For this reason, it pays to become sun-conscious, and to plan your activities according to the time of day. For instance, during the summer, try to run errands and engage in outdoor activities early in the morning or late in the afternoon, rather than running around at high noon.

Whether you choose to shield the backs of your hands with a hand cream that contains sunscreen or with a plain sunscreen, be sure that the product you use has an SPF of at least 15—the minimum sun protection factor recommended by experts. If you have fair skin, you might consider using a sunscreen with a higher SPF. High SPF sunscreens can be irritating to your skin, though, so if your hands feel itchy, warm, or sore after using a product with a high SPF, scale back to an SPF of 15.

Just as important as applying a sunscreen when you first go outdoors is *reapplying* it often. Research shows that frequent reapplication of a sunscreen with a moderate SPF may be more effective than a single application of a high-SPF sunscreen. By applying your sunscreen frequently, you will be sure that it's on your skin and working. Sunscreens can wear off pretty quickly, depending on what you're doing. For easy on-the-go application, buy one of the many sunscreens now available in stick form. These are small and won't spill, so that you can carry one in your purse. Just as important, the stick form enables you to apply the product to the back of your hand without getting it on the palm of your hand. (Sunscreen that remains on the palm can be easily rubbed into your eyes or transferred to the foods you're eating.) If you have no sunscreen on hand, and you find yourself outdoors, feel free to use a lip balm that contains sunscreen.

Last, don't forget that exposing unprotected skin to the sun can cause more than just wrinkles and brown spots. It can lead to skin cancer, a potentially dangerous condition. So don't spare the sunscreen! (To learn more about skin cancer and other disorders that can affect the skin, see the inset on page 96.)

Recognizing Skin- and Hand-Related Disorders

A number of disorders can alter the appearance of your hand, either by affecting the skin or by affecting underlying structures. In addition, they can cause varying degrees of discomfort and, in some cases, may have more serious consequences. It is important to recognize these disorders so that you can seek appropriate professional help. This inset briefly examines four of the most common disorders that can affect the appearance and well-being of your skin and hands.

Dermatitis

Dermatitis—also called eczema—is an inflammation of the skin that produces scaling, flaking, thickening, color changes, and itching or pain. One of the most common types of dermatitis is *contact dermatitis*, an allergic reaction resulting from contact with perfumes, cosmetics, rubber, medicated creams and ointments, metals such as nickel, or other allergens. Many health care workers have been found to have an allergy to the latex gloves they wear to perform their work. Whatever the irritant, as long as you remain in contact with it, the condition is likely to spread and become more severe.

If you seem to have the symptoms of contact dermatitis and you don't know the source of the problem, see your dermatologist as soon as possible. A doctor can help you identify the allergen as well as other products that might trigger an allergic reaction. He or she may recommend that you avoid repeated wetting of the hands by wearing rubber gloves while washing dishes, for instance, and may also be able to prescribe a medication that will alleviate your symptoms.

Warts

Those warts that occur on the hands are usually *common warts*. Like all warts, these are caused by a virus. Common warts usually have a rough surface; are gray, yellow, or brown in color; and may be round or irregular in shape. They may appear singly or in clusters.

Although warts are benign and harmless, and typically do not cause pain or itching, they are contagious, and may be spread if they are picked, trimmed, bitten, or touched. For this reason, it is important to avoid picking or cutting a wart, and to see a dermatologist as soon as possible if you know or suspect that you have one. Your doctor can remove warts using a variety of methods.

Arthritis

Arthritis is an inflammation of the joints characterized by pain, swelling, stiffness, and diminished range of motion. When the hands are affected, knuckles and other joints may become deformed and enlarged. There are several types of arthritis, including rheumatoid arthritis, osteoarthritis, and psoriatic arthritis. Each has its own causes and may result in symptoms other than the most common ones listed above.

If you are suffering from arthritis, it is important to seek medical attention. Your doctor may be able to prescribe medications, physical therapy, diet, or other treatments that can alleviate pain and perhaps avoid further distortion of the joints.

Skin Cancer

Of the many types of skin cancer that exist, the major ones most likely to affect your hands are squamous cell carcinoma and melanoma.

Squamous cell carcinoma begins in the middle layer of the epidermis. (See page 20 for a look at the anatomy of the skin.) Often the result of sun damage, it first appears as a red area with a scaly, crusted surface. As it grows, a firm tumor develops, sometimes resembling a wart or a small ulcerated spot that doesn't heal.

Melanoma is less common than squamous cell carcinoma, but more serious. In this condition, a tumor arises from the pigment-producing cells of the epidermis. Most melanomas form flat dark patches on the skin. It is estimated that nearly half of all cases originate in moles. If not treated at an early stage, melanoma can spread through the bloodstream and lymph vessels to the internal organs, and can be life threatening.

Although some types of skin cancer are more serious than others, *all* should be treated promptly. For this reason, it is important to be aware of any new growth on the skin of your hands or of any other part of your body; of an open sore that bleeds, crusts over, but does not heal properly; or of a change in a mole. Any of these may indicate the presence of a cancer, and should be promptly brought to your doctor's attention. Remember that skin cancer is treatable, but recovery depends on early detection.

REHABILITATION FOR HANDS

If you've been using your Beautiful Hands and Nails Regimen, your hands may be smoother and softer than they've been in a long time. Still, years of sun, wind, detergents, and the like have probably taken their toll, and your hands may need additional help. The remainder of this chapter will provide you with just that. First, you'll find a myriad of treatments designed to smooth, soothe, and soften rough, dry, chapped hands. Following this you'll find treatments that can help you banish those nasty brown spots. You'll even learn how to thoroughly clean hands that have become extra-grimy—without harming your skin. And a special inset will tell you about some "emergency" hand-care techniques that will allow you to clean, smooth, and soothe your hands in only one session.

Smoothing and Softening Your Hands

If you are plagued by rough, dry hands—hands that snag delicate fabrics and tear pantyhose—you'll be delighted by the following treatments. They smooth, they soothe, and they soften, and best of all, they do it *without oiliness.* Use these treatments often, always reapplying your nail protector and hand cream directly afterwards. You will be rewarded by softer, more beautiful hands.

Bran Hand Softener

This old-fashioned treatment is a very effective nongreasy skin softener that will make your hands feel like silk. The treatment is particularly enjoyable on a cold day or whenever your hands feel achy.

Simply place a cup of boiling water in a large heatproof bowl, and mix in a half cup of bran. Allow the mixture to cool off just until it is comfortably warm. Then immerse your hands and wash them with the bran for three or four minutes.

Finally, rinse your hands with warm water, and dry them thoroughly. Use this treatment as often as desired.

Lavender Hand Water

Cosmetic vinegars have been used for centuries to make skin soft and fragrant. Use Lavender Hand Water whenever your skin becomes rough and chapped, or when it retains the odor of garlic and onions.

To make Lavender Hand Water, ideally, you'll want to use a small bundle of fresh lavender, a few sprigs of fresh rosemary and thyme, and a rose geranium leaf. If you don't have access to fresh herbs, though, just substitute a quarter cup of dried lavender, and a teaspoon each of rosemary and thyme. (Leave out the rose geranium.) Place the herbs in a clean one-quart mayonnaise jar. If fresh herbs are being used, the jar should be just about full of loosely packed leaves. Add white vinegar to fill the jar, cover, and place in the sun, either outside or on a windowsill. Allow to sit for three or four days, shaking the mixture daily.

When ready, strain the mixture through a sieve into a pretty jar. To use, add a tablespoon of Lavender Hand Water to a bowl of warm water, and use it to rinse your hands as often as desired.

Egg White Hand Mask

The protein in the Egg White Hand Mask will soothe your chapped skin, leaving your hands smooth and soft.

To benefit from this unusual treatment, simply separate an egg, allowing the white to drop onto a dinner plate. (Reserve the yolk for another use.) Place one hand on the plate, and rub the white briskly over the skin. Be sure to massage the egg white into the fingers and the back of the hand. The egg will get slightly "whipped up," turning a frothy white. Change hands, and continue for one or two minutes. Then rinse your hands well with warm water and dry them thoroughly. Use the mask as often as desired.

Oatmeal Softening Treatment

This easy-to-prepare mask is a great way to make your hands feel smooth and satiny. And it's so mild that you can use it as a facial mask, too!

To make Oatmeal Softening Treatment, place a little over a quarter cup of organic oatmeal in a blender, and blend until finely ground. You should have a quarter cup. (Adjust the amount if necessary.) Place the ground meal in a large bowl, add a tablespoon of spring water or aloe vera juice, and mix well.

Rub the oatmeal mixture all over your hands, massaging it in well. Be sure to massage your wrists and your fingers, including your knuckles and cuticles. After three to five minutes of rubbing, rinse well with warm water and dry your hands thoroughly. Use this treatment as often as desired.

Cornmeal and Olive Oil Exfoliating Treatment

Normally, you shouldn't use any exfoliating treatment on the hands, as the skin on the back of the hands is paper thin. This soft, oily mixture, though, is a gentle way to make your skin feel like velvet and, as a bonus, to leave your hands invigorated and tingling.

Place a quarter cup of cornmeal, two tablespoons of vegetable oil, and, if desired, the contents of a vitamin E capsule in a large bowl, and mix. Holding your hands over the bowl, rub the mixture over your hands, gently massaging each finger, cuticle, and knuckle, as well as the wrists. Pay special attention to any brown spots. Continue to rub gently for a few more minutes. Then wash your hands thoroughly with mild castile soap, rinse, and dry. Repeat this treatment as often as once a week.

Simple Papaya Hand Treatment

The enzymes in papayas are great for loosening the dead cells found on the skin's surface, and revealing the smooth skin beneath. Since enzymes are strong, avoid using this treatment if your skin is very sensitive, your cuticles are torn, or you have dermatitis.

To make Simple Papaya Hand Treatment, mash a small piece of ripe papaya until you have about a tablespoon of smooth pulp. Then massage the pulp over your hands and well into your cuticles. Allow the pulp to remain on your hands for a minute or so; then rinse well. Use this treatment as often as every other week.

Intensive Moisturizing Treatment

When temperatures plummet, hands can quickly become dry, chapped, and painful. They may even crack and bleed. Intensive Moisturizing Treatment is the perfect therapy for hands that need relief from the abuses of winter weather.

Simply stir together one tablespoon of lanolin and one tablespoon of petroleum jelly until well mixed. Then apply just enough of the mixture to your hands to form a thin coat. Massage the mixture in thoroughly, paying special attention to the cuticles and knuckles.

Leave the mixture on for about twenty minutes, allowing the warmth of your hands to melt the ingredients so that they can penetrate the skin. Then, using a mild liquid castile soap, wash your hands under warm running water. It will take two or three latherings to remove the treatment mixture. What will remain is a very thin protective film that is not at all greasy. During the coldest months, you may want to use this treatment once a week.

The White Glove Treatment

This is another wonderful treatment for red, cracked, painful hands—in other words, hands that are urgently in need of help. The gloves give the fats in the petroleum jelly "dressing" a chance to penetrate your skin, providing your hands with speedy relief and helping to promote healing.

Intensive Care for Hands

This chapter presents a variety of natural treatments that can help soften and smooth your hands. They are meant to be used periodically, in addition to your Beautiful Hands and Nails Regimen, to help keep hands at their best. But what if you have really let your hands go? Perhaps you went on a gardening spree—without your gloves. Or maybe you refinished furniture or cleaned the garage. *And* you've been neglecting your four-part regimen. (For shame!) The result? Your hands look like they belong to a lumberjack. Is there any way you can rehabilitate them quickly, removing days—perhaps weeks!—of accumulated grime, hard cuticles, and roughened skin? Of course there is!

Emergency Hand Rehabilitation

This treatment combines a series of proven techniques designed to gently but thoroughly clean, soften, and exfoliate hands, cuticles, and nails in a single treatment. It takes a while—about an hour. But it's worth it!

Small bar of soap, such as Ivory
3 teaspoons baking soda
½ teaspoon 3-percent hydrogen peroxide
1 tablespoon cornmeal
1 vitamin E capsule
Petroleum jelly
Mild liquid castile soap

Several small bowls
Natural bristle nail brush
Pumice stone
Plastic gloves
Small towel

1. Place the bar of soap in a small dish, and cover it with water. Set aside for 5 minutes.

2. Place the baking soda and hydrogen peroxide in a small bowl, and stir to mix. Set aside.

3. Place the cornmeal in another small bowl, and set aside.

4. Prick the vitamin E capsule with a pin, and set aside.

5. Scrape your nails over the softened soap. Be sure to get the soap under the entire nail, both at the tip of the finger and on the sides. Remove the soap from the water, reserving the soapy liquid. If your nails are extremely grimy, leave the soap under them for at least 15 minutes before proceeding to the next step. If not, immediately proceed.

6. With the soap still under your fingernails, thoroughly massage the nail and cuticle with some of the cornmeal, taking your time to exfoliate and clean the cuticles.

7. Under running water, use your nail brush to remove all of the cornmeal and soap from under the nail. Dry your hands well.

8. Using your fingers or a cotton swab, pack the baking soda mixture under the nails. Leave in place for at least 5 minutes; leave on longer if the nails are yellowed or grimy. Again, use a nail brush to remove the mixture.

9. Use the pumice stone to smooth any calluses on your fingers. Don't try to totally remove the calluses; just smooth them and remove any flaky, dead skin. Dry your hands well.

10. Squeeze a drop of vitamin E oil on each nail, and massage it into the cuticles. Then massage a *very* small amount of petroleum jelly all over your hands, and put on the plastic gloves. Leave on for 30 minutes—longer, if possible.

11. Pour a little of the reserved soap water into the remaining cornmeal, and massage the mixture over the nail and cuticle. Rinse well. Then use the castile soap and nail brush to remove every particle of the cornmeal. Dry your hands well, pushing back the cuticles with the towel. And you're done!

The Fifteen-Minute Hand Revamp

This treatment will make your hands just a little bit smoother and softer, and your nails just a little bit whiter. And if your hands have become unpleasantly dry, it will make them more comfortable, too. The Hand Revamp is just the thing when you don't have time for Emergency Hand Rehabilitation—or your hands really aren't bad enough to warrant a long procedure—but you feel that you need a quick lift.

---

1 tablespoon regular or low-fat plain yogurt
Natural bristle nail brush
Nail-whitening pencil
Nail file
Lanolin
Hand cream

1. Smooth the yogurt over your hands and lower arms. Allow it to remain in place for 2 to 3 minutes. Then rinse well with warm water. Using your nail brush, brush your hands and nails very briefly to remove any remaining yogurt.

2. While your hands and nails are still damp, pass a nail-whitening pencil briefly under each nail tip. (These pencils work best when nails are still a bit moist.)

3. Dry your hands thoroughly. If any nails need smoothing or reshaping, touch up quickly with the file.

4. Place a tiny dab of lanolin on each nail, and massage it in. Rub in some hand cream, and you're done!

Apply a thin layer of petroleum jelly to your hands and nails. Using a tissue, put on first one plastic glove, and then the other. (Use the thin gloves sold in hardware stores.) Now watch TV or nap for at least half an hour. When the time is up, remove the gloves and wash your hands with your mild castile soap. Lather and rinse two or three times, depending on the amount of petroleum jelly used. Stop sudsing when only a slight film still remains. Dry your hands with a soft terry cloth towel, pushing back the cuticles. Your hands will feel much more comfortable. Because this treatment is so gentle, feel free to use it whenever you have the time.

Warm Paraffin Hand Treatment

The Warm Paraffin Hand Treatment is an effective hand and cuticle softener. It is also a soothing treatment, perfect for use on arthritic hands.

Chop half a pound of paraffin into small pieces, and place

in a shallow heatproof bowl or a Pyrex pie plate. (You can find paraffin in the canning supplies section of your supermarket or in a hobby supplies store.) If desired, add a teaspoon of vitamin E oil. Pour an inch of water into a twelve-inch skillet, and place the dish of paraffin in the skillet. Place over low heat until melted. Remember that paraffin is flammable, so keep your eye on the skillet!

Once the wax is melted, remove it from the heat and allow to cool for about fifteen minutes. Then carefully test it with a fingertip to see if it is just comfortably warm. Don't use it while it's hot, or you can cause a serious burn!

Thoroughly wash your hands prior to treatment. If you're treating your entire hand, place one hand at a time in the melted wax, turning to coat both sides. Remember to coat your wrists, too. If you suffer from cracked fingertips, you may, if you prefer, dip just your fingertips into the warm paraffin.

Allow the wax to remain on your hands for at least fifteen minutes, or until completely cool. Then simply crumble off the paraffin, and return it to the pie pan. (You can reuse the wax many times.) Use this treatment as often as desired.

Banishing "Age" Spots

If you've ever thought that no simple home remedy can fade those annoying age spots, think again. While I know of no natural techniques that will *instantly* make spots vanish, there are a number of easy-to-use treatments that can gradually fade these spots—*if* you use them faithfully. In this case, persistence is the key to success.

When treating age spots, it's important to remember that they're really not caused by age. And although they're sometimes referred to as liver spots, they're not caused by liver problems, either. Rather, these flat brown spots are the result of damage caused by excessive exposure to the sun. Therefore, both throughout treatment and afterwards, it is vital that you *keep using your sunscreen!* Without it, spots will darken and worsen with time.

As you use the following treatments, keep in mind that most of these "recipes" will yield enough for several treatments. Store leftovers in a covered container in the refrigerator, and use them as soon as possible.

Lemon Buttermilk Hand Bleach

This old-fashioned skin bleach—Scarlett O'Hara was fond of buttermilk bleaches—has been revamped to make use of dried buttermilk powder. You can find this product in the baking section of your supermarket.

Mix a tablespoon of the buttermilk powder with a tablespoon of fresh lemon juice and a few drops of vitamin E oil. Pat the mixture over the backs of your hands, making sure that all brown spots are covered. Allow the mixture to remain in place for at least thirty minutes; then rinse thoroughly with warm water. Use this treatment as often as once a week on skin of normal sensitivity, and as often as every other week for sensitive skin.

Barley Flour Hand Bleach

The use of barley flour to smooth hands and feet dates back to ancient Babylon. Just as important, I've found that this wonderful flour can gradually fade age spots.

Mix about a quarter cup of barley flour with an equal amount of water, and stir for about thirty seconds to a minute—long enough to allow the mixture to thicken to a paste. Apply the paste to the backs of your hands, and allow it to remain in place for five to ten minutes. Then rinse your hands thoroughly, and dry. Use this treatment as often as desired.

Potato Peel Hand Pack

This amazingly simple hand pack will smooth your skin and *slightly* lighten any spots—but sometimes, that slight lightening is all you need. Just be aware that some people are allergic to raw potato juice, so try a peel or two before applying the whole treatment.

Nothing could be simpler than this pack. Apply a handful of potato peels, one at a time, to the backs of your hand, with the cut sides against your skin. Leave each peel in place for up to a minute. Then rinse your hands and dry them. Your hands will feel cool and refreshed. Use this treatment as often as desired.

Avocado Peel Pack

Believe it or not, in addition to being delicious, avocados can help fade age spots. And it couldn't be easier to use them!

Simply smooth the inside of an avocado peel over the backs of your hands, paying particular attention to the brown spots. Allow the oils to sink in for about ten minutes; then rinse lightly to remove any excess oil. Use as often as desired. (By the way, if you don't have time for this treatment right after peeling your avocado, simply keep the peels sealed in the freezer until needed.)

Lemon and Oats Lightener

This treatment will fade spots *and* smooth skin at the same time.

Place two tablespoons of oatmeal in a blender, and blend until it has the consistency of a powder. Place the powder in a small dish, and mix in a tablespoon of lemon juice until a paste is formed. Massage the paste into the spots on the back of your hands, allowing the mixture to remain in place for a minute or two. Then rinse well and dry. Use as often as desired.

Alpha-Hydroxy Acid Treatments

So far, we've discussed treatments that smooth and moisturize hands, and treatments that fade age spots. Alpha-hydroxy acids (AHAs) not only perform both these functions, but do so in a unique way. These acids loosen dead skin cells from the skin's surface, allowing them to be sloughed off. This, in turn, stimulates new skin cell production, enabling newer, fresher skin to emerge. When used on sun-damaged skin, AHAs also reduce discoloration and even out pigmentation.

You are probably aware that AHAs are now available in many commercial products. What you may *not* know is that they naturally occur in buttermilk, yogurt, honey, berries, citrus fruits, apples, avocados, corn, and a host of other foods. The beauty of using these foods in your treatments lies in their safety, simplicity, and effectiveness.

If you have never used an alpha-hydroxy acid treatment, don't let the word "acid" scare you. The pH of these substances is on the acid side—about 3.0 to 4.5—but they are acidic only in the sense that a tomato or sour apple is acidic. Nevertheless, be aware that it is normal for these treatments to cause a little stinging sensation, especially if your hands have tiny cuts or abrasions. However, a pronounced uncomfortable stinging may mean that your skin is too sensitive for these treatments.

One last point—when using the following treatments, don't forget your wrists. A bracelet of lines can encircle your wrists as you grow older. By gently rubbing these treatments into your wrists, you'll keep these lines to a minimum.

Yogurt Smoother

This treatment will leave your skin wonderfully soft. And on a hot day, when your hands feel warm and swollen, the cold yogurt will also have a delightfully cooling effect.

Simply hold your hands over a dinner plate or sink, and smooth a tablespoon or so of regular or low-fat plain yogurt over your hands, wrists, and lower arms. Allow the yogurt to remain in place for two to three minutes. Then rinse thoroughly and dry. Use as often as needed.

If desired, you can customize this smoother by adding a few drops of essential oil to each treatment. Lavender oil and chamomile oil are both good choices. You can also combine yogurt with other AHA-containing substances, as follows:

❑ To make Yogurt and Lemon Smoother, combine the juice of one lemon with eight ounces of regular or low-fat plain yogurt. Cover and chill for several hours to allow the mixture to mellow. Then use as you would Yogurt Smoother. Refrigerate any leftovers for up to two weeks.

❑ To make Yogurt and Honey Smoother, mix a tablespoon of regular or low-fat plain yogurt with a tablespoon of honey. Use as you would Yogurt Smoother.

Avocado and Honey Smoother

This delightfully creamy treatment will provide you with AHAs from two different sources. Just peel and mash half of a very ripe avocado with one tablespoon of honey until smooth and creamy. Slather the mixture over your hands and wrists, and leave in place for five minutes. Rinse thoroughly and dry. Use as often as desired.

Honey and Lemon Smoother

Thoroughly mix a tablespoon of honey with the juice of half a fresh lemon. Massage the mixture into your hands for several minutes. Then rinse thoroughly, dry, and enjoy soft hands! Use as often as desired.

Buttermilk Smoother

For many years, Southern belles rubbed buttermilk over their hands and arms to fade freckles and smooth their skin. You can do the same today. Or, if you prefer, make a buttermilk-fruit treatment by mashing some berries—raspberries or strawberries, for instance—and mixing them with the buttermilk. Use as often as desired.

Gently Cleaning *Really* Dirty Hands

Your Beautiful Hands and Nails Regimen will help keep your hands clean and soft. Sometimes, though, hands get extra-dirty, and need extra attention. And although there are products on the market that are designed to clean grimy hands, they tend to be harsh. Below, you will find my method for cleaning hands of ground-in dirt both effectively and gently. Following that, I present my recipe for a wonderfully gentle nonsoap cleanser that you may prefer to commercially available products.

Fast Cornmeal Hand Scrub

This is a simple, mild, yet highly effective way to clean hands that have become grimy through yard work, arts and crafts projects, or what have you. First, wash your hands well with mild liquid castile soap or unscented glycerin soap. While your hands are still covered with lather, use a tablespoon of cornmeal to gently scrub any especially dirty areas, such as calluses. Cornmeal is very gentle, so feel free to scrub briskly. If your hands are still stained, rub a small amount of soap into the grimy areas and allow the soap to dissolve the dirt for a minute or two. Then use your nail brush to scrub off the soap. If your hands are *still* stained, try rubbing a piece of fresh lemon peel over the dirty areas.

Fluffy Cleanser

While mild castile and glycerin soaps are good cleansers, I often use one of my own invention—Fluffy Cleanser—to clean hands that are especially dirty or stained, or that have a persistent odor from cooking with fish, onions, or garlic. To make this mild nonsoap cleanser, simply mix together equal parts of baking soda, nonfat dry milk powder, and cornstarch. Store the mixture in a small plastic container, and keep it in your bathroom or kitchen. To use, wet your hands and sprinkle them with a tablespoon or less of the cleanser. As you wash, the baking soda will make the cleanser foam up a bit. Then rinse. Your hands will be left clean, soft, soothed, and odorless.

You can easily customize Fluffy Cleanser to meet your own needs. If you have dermatitis, try increasing the proportion of cornstarch to make the cleanser even more soothing. If your hands are extremely sensitive, try leaving out the baking soda entirely. And if you cook with onions and garlic almost every day, increase the amount of baking soda.

REHABILITATION FOR ARMS

Because hands so quickly show signs of abuse, we tend to focus on them at the expense of our arms. But over time, even your arms will begin to sport age spots and other signs of wear. Considering that, visually, hands and arms are a cohesive unit, a little attention to arms is definitely worth your while.

Let's start with the upper arms, which can sometimes be plagued by bumpy skin. Fortunately, nothing fancy is needed to solve this problem. As often as possible, use a loofah sponge or natural bristle body brush to scrub this area, sloughing off dead cells and smoothing the skin.

Moving down, we reach the elbows—one of the most neglected areas of the body. The skin covering the elbows is thicker than that on the rest of the arm, and when dry skin cells build up, the elbows can look dark and scruffy. The solution? Every day, cream your elbows directly after your bath or shower, while your skin is still slightly moist. At least once a week, use a loofah sponge and a mild liquid castile or unscented glycerin soap on your elbows. Finally, once a month, massage each elbow with a handful of cornmeal. This consistent, gentle care will keep your elbows smooth and attractive.

Finally, we reach the lower arm. The best way to smooth the lower arms, along with the hands and, if you like, the upper arms, is to alternate use of the Yogurt and Lemon Smoother (page 109) with that of the Hand and Arm De-Ager (see below). This easy one-two punch will smooth and soften hands and arms like nothing else.

Hand and Arm De-Ager

The results of this treatment will surprise you. Your hands and arms will be noticeably smoother and softer, with none of the greasy feeling that moisturizers often leave behind.

Place about two tablespoons of glycerin and two tablespoons of 3-percent hydrogen peroxide in a glass cup or bowl. Holding your hands over a dinner plate or the bathroom sink, pour the mixture over your hands, and smooth the mixture over your hands, wrists, and arms. Massage it into your skin for a minute or two; then rinse well with warm water and dry thoroughly.

PREVENTION: THE KEY TO YOUNGER-LOOKING HANDS

Now that you've learned how to smooth your hands and arms, as well as how to fade those dreadful age spots, we return to the theme with which our chapter began—prevention. Especially as you get older, any damage caused by exposure to the sun, by harsh chemicals, or by other types of abuse becomes harder and harder to repair. It's so much simpler to avoid this damage to begin with. And it's so easy to do so by protecting your hands with the appropriate gloves and by using sunscreen whenever you go outdoors. This is the best beautiful-hands strategy of all.

Chapter 7

Healthy Habits for Beautiful Hands and Nails

Healthy nails are naturally beautiful. They are as smooth as the inside of a seashell, as delicate as a rose petal. The nail itself is translucent and evenly textured, not cloudy, thickened, rippled, or whitened. The nail bed is evenly colored, and the cuticle protecting the nail is smooth and elastic, not rough and hard. The nail tips are an even white or light ivory, not yellow or unevenly stained. And when these nails appear on smooth, well-cared-for hands, they add so much to your overall appearance!

In previous chapters, you have seen how a simple four-part routine and some easy-to-use treatments can help restore the health and enhance the appearance of your nails and hands. But it's important to remember that the health of your nails and skin is a direct result of your *overall* well-being—which is why so many doctors begin a physical examination by looking at a patient's hands. Pale nail beds; a pitted nail surface; and dull, lifeless skin can be red flags indicating nutritional deficiencies, inadequate exercise, inadequate rest, smoking, and other poor lifestyle habits. Skin and nails that radiate health reflect a healthful lifestyle as well as good nail and hand care.

In Chapter 6, you learned about the most common hazards that everyday life poses to the delicate skin on your hands. In this chapter, you'll learn about specific disorders, habits, and substances that can cause your nails to become "sick." You'll then learn about some simple lifestyle changes—changes like improved diet and increased exercise—that can promote general well-being and, in the process, help make both your nails *and* your hands glowingly healthy.

HOW NAILS GET SICK

Composed of layers of dead cells, nails themselves don't actually get sick. But substances applied to the nail, often in the name of improved nail appearance and strength, can irritate the tissue around the nail, making the nail itself look unhealthy. In addition, poor general health—as well as specific lifestyle practices, such as smoking—can cause discolored nail beds, compromised strength, and a variety of other nail problems.

How Nails Mirror Health Problems

Many serious medical conditions can manifest themselves through nail abnormalities. Very pale nail beds sometimes indicate anemia, while bluish nail beds can indicate heart or lung problems; in all of these instances, your body is providing your extremities with insufficient oxygen. Kidney, thyroid, liver, and pituitary gland problems also can reveal themselves through abnormal nail bed color. Severe arthritis that inflames the finger joints can lead to nail splitting, and tiny pits in the nails can indicate psoriasis.

In each of these cases, professional help should be sought to deal with the underlying problem. Often, once proper medical care is received—for instance, when iron supplements are used to treat anemia—the resulting nail problem is eliminated.

Another Reason to Quit Smoking

No discussion of nail health—or of health in general—can be complete without at least a brief look at smoking. True, smoking doesn't affect your nails in the immediate, obvious way that nail biting or a fungal infection can harm them. But its effects are no less real.

How does smoking affect your nails? Your nails are loaded with capillaries—tiny blood vessels that carry oxygenated blood to the nail bed. The nicotine in the cigarette constricts these vessels, depleting the oxygen that travels to the nail bed and the nail-generating matrix. The oxygen-deprived nail beds become pasty and leaden in appearance, and the nails can grow more slowly, almost reluctantly. If that wasn't bad enough, nicotine stains the fingertips and makes the hands smell of stale smoke. Not a pretty picture, is it?

True, nail health isn't the number-one reason cited to quit smoking. But when you think of what smoking is doing to your nails and your hands, you can imagine what it's doing to the rest of your body. So for the health of your entire body, give up smoking. Your nails will thank you!

Fungal Infections

Fungal infections of the nails are a fairly common problem. Under certain circumstances, fungal spores attach themselves to the cells of the nail, digesting the keratin and setting up house inside the cells. When such an infection occurs, the affected nails become thickened, discolored, and crumbly. This infection can begin on one part of the nail—on the tip of the nail or the new cells at the base of the nail, for instance—and work its way through the remainder of the nail. Over time, the infection can travel from nail to nail, and can even be transmitted to another person. Ultimately, the fungus can cause the nail to separate from the nail bed below it, and the nail can be lost.

Artificial Nails

It wasn't that long ago that only a few women wore artificial nails, and most of these women were glamorous models or flamboyant film personalities. As late as the 1960s and 1970s, it was necessary to have a manicurist apply the nails through a somewhat lengthy procedure. Today, though, beauty supply stores, drugstores, and even supermarkets offer a bounty of do-it-yourself products that allow women to apply artificial nails at home. In fact, the majority of the nail-care products sold today are designed to create and maintain artificial nails. Admittedly, these nails can be as hard as iron, and can seem a quick route to nail glamour. But they can also be a quick route to real nail problems.

The first problem occurs when women nervously peel the tips of the fake nails off, and consequently peel off the top layer of the *real* nail beneath. This leaves the real nail thin and weakened.

A more serious problem occurs as the real nail grows out and the artificial nail moves down, leaving a "naked" area between the cuticle and the top of the fake nail. When water seeps into this gap and under the artificial nail, the stage is set for fungal growth. And as you learned in the discussion on page 115, if the fungal growth is allowed to continue unchecked, the *real* nail can be lost to such an infection. If you doubt the connection between artificial nail use and fungal infections, take a tour of your local drugstore. Very often, you'll find that remedies for nail fungus are sold *next* to the artificial nail products.

The bottom line is that artificial nails spell trouble, and should be avoided. Instead, protect your nails with natural products and nourish them from the inside instead of burdening them with polymer straightjackets. Baby them, and they'll repay you by being healthy, resilient, and beautiful!

What causes fungal nail infections? One of the most common causes is the use of artificial nails. These nails can trap moisture beneath them, leading to fungal growth. (To learn more about the problems caused by artificial nails, see the inset above.) But you don't have to use artificial nails to have this problem. If your nails become soaked with water while washing dishes or taking a bath, and you subsequently apply a coat of nail enamel without first allowing the nails to dry out, you will seal in the dampness, setting the stage for fungal infection. You might not even realize what's happening until you remove the polish and see the patches of crumbling white or yellowish nail beneath. In addition, fungal infections can be transmitted from person to person through the use of shared manicure tools. In fact, the growing popularity of nail salons has caused the incidence of fungal nail infections to increase, as infections get passed from patron to patron. Ideally, either the nail-care tools should be sterilized between uses, or each patron should carry her own set of tools that are used only on her.

If you notice the beginning of a fungal infection on your nails, try soaking them in 3-percent hydrogen peroxide for one to two minutes, a few times a day. A potent antifungal compound, hydrogen peroxide is easily absorbed by the nails. You can also try applications of tea tree oil, another natural antifungal agent. But if your home remedies don't bring improvement within two to four days, make a beeline for your dermatologist.

Nail-Care Products

It is ironic that products designed to make your nails look beautiful and enhance their strength can actually *harm* your nails. But it's true. Earlier in the chapter, you learned how artificial nails and even nail polish can lead to fungal growth. But other products can cause other types of problems.

Like any type of cosmetic substance, nail-care products have the potential to cause allergic reactions. For instance, chemical substances such as formaldehyde, which is found in many hardeners, can cause a rash in the skin around the nail, or may cause the nail to begin separating from the nail bed. To make matters worse, formaldehyde "hardens" nails by dehydrating them—a process that can lead to brittleness and subsequent nail breakage. Of course, you can simply avoid products that list formaldehyde as an ingredient. Keep in mind, though, that this isn't always as easy as it sounds. Recently I saw a new nail hardener at my local pharmacy. Its secret ingredient? Mathenol. What was that, I wondered. The ingredients list yielded the answer—mathenol is formaldehyde!

The solvents and glues found in artificial nail products can also cause rashes in some women. And while some products may not directly hurt the nail, they can hurt *you*. For instance, toluene, a lacquer solvent used in nail polish, has been found to enter the body through the nails and lead to symptoms such as dizziness and mental confusion. While many major cosmetic companies have discontinued use of this substance, it is not illegal, and may still be found in some products.

Of course, the solution to the problem of harmful nail-care products is simple—use only *natural* products to shine, color, and strengthen your nails. By following your four-step regimen and using only the treatments presented in this book, you can have beautiful nails without using potentially harmful chemicals.

Nail Biting

Perhaps one of the most common practices that can damage your nails is nail biting. And while it may seem like a harmless though unattractive habit, nail biting can actually result in more than just nail damage. People who bite their nails to the point of bleeding—and perhaps bite their cuticles, too—can end up with potentially serious infections that require medical attention.

Of course, most nail biting doesn't reach this point. If you bite your nails just enough to sabotage your efforts to have pretty nails, there are easy steps you can take to eliminate this habit. (See the inset on page 120.) If, however, you consistently bite your nails down to the quick, it would be wise to seek help from a physician, a therapist, or another professional who can uncover the cause of this behavior and help you rid yourself of the habit.

LIFESTYLE CHANGES FOR HEALTHY HANDS AND NAILS

I don't know about you, but I am glad to see the end of our discussion of "sick" nails, and eager to think about nails that are rosy with health. As I've already discussed, such nails are not the product of good nail care only. They also require good food, proper exercise, sufficient rest—everything that is needed for good *general* health. And, fortunately, what's good for your nails is also good for your hands. In the remainder of this chapter, we'll examine each of these components of a nail- and hand-healthy lifestyle.

Getting a Good Night's Sleep

Years ago, I never would have begun a discussion of nail and skin health with the subject of sleep. Perhaps it's obvious that good nutrition and grooming are necessary for beautiful hands—but sleep? Yet the more I learn about the human body, the more I know that good-quality sleep is crucial to having great-looking nails and hands.

How does sleep help your skin and nails? Ideally, you drift off to dreamland within minutes of your head hitting the pillow. As you dream, your body is very busy, because it has to repair all of the damage that occurred that day. About an hour after you fall asleep, an elevated level of growth and repair hormones begins to circulate everywhere throughout the body, including the capillary-rich nail beds and the basal layer of the epidermis, where new skin cells are produced. While it is not known precisely how these hormones function, they do seem to play a role in boosting cellular growth and in repairing or destroying damaged cells.

One other wonderful thing happens when you sleep. You relax deeply. Not just your muscles relax, but also your blood vessels. As a result, the vessels expand, allowing increased blood flow to your hands, feet, and face.

Nail Biting—An Effective Plan to Kick the Habit

Nail biting is an all-too-common habit. And anyone who practices it can tell you that no matter how much you hate what it does to your nails, it is a difficult habit to break. But even if you have been biting your nails for years, you'll be glad to know that there are a few simple steps that can help you stop biting, and start enjoying the pleasures of beautiful hands and nails. Here they are:

❏ Neglected, rough, ragged nails and cuticles can serve as a magnet for nail biting. So, most important, start your Beautiful Hands and Nails Regimen, and follow it faithfully. Apply white iodine to any inflamed areas of the cuticle. It will sting slightly, but it will also help heal any inflammation. Then make Calendula Cuticle Salve (page 57), and use it to heal hangnails and any bitten areas around the nails. Use my natural exfoliants to smooth your cuticles, and your hand cream to baby your hands. File your nails carefully as they grow out. Believe it or not, you'll find that as your nails and cuticles become smoother and more attractive, you will bite them less. In fact, after a while, there won't be anything to bite—no jagged nail edges, no ragged cuticles. Just as important, this will bolster your self-esteem and give you greater incentive to respect your nails. Gradually, the nail-biting habit will fade.

❏ Instead of telling yourself to stop biting your nails—a strategy that tends to meet with limited success—simply try to keep your hands away from your face. Nail biters also tend to fidget with their hair, scratch their heads, and rub their chins. So concentrate on keeping your hands either in repose or engaged in some sort of task, and you'll bite less.

❏ Consider the situations that trigger your nail biting. It might be something as trivial as being stuck in traffic; or it could be a job or a relationship that causes you to be tense. Then the next time you are in the "trigger" situation, consciously keep your hands folded in your lap or busy doing something else. Awareness of your triggers can be a tremendous help in breaking your habit.

❏ Try rubbing a dab of myrrh oil into each nail tip. Although myrrh oil smells wonderful, it is bitter in taste. This oil is a safe way to discourage biting. (To learn more about myrrh oil, see page 83.)

❑ Help rid yourself of anxiety and tension by taking a few moments for a "time out" each and every day. Stop worrying—tell yourself that you can begin worrying again as soon as your break is over!—and have a soothing cup of tea. Sage tea, a tea long used as a "nerve tonic," is a particularly good aid to relaxation. Simply place three fresh sage leaves (or one tablespoon of dried leaves) in your most beautiful china teacup, and pour boiling water over the leaves. Cover the cup with a saucer and allow to steep for at least ten minutes. Then contemplate the leaves as they float in the tea, and sip appreciatively.

Finally, allow yourself to fail occasionally. If you have been biting your nails for years, you will have to learn what it feels like *not* to bite them. Your hands were previously the focus of your attention. Now you have to gradually learn to allow your nails to heal and grow. As you care for your nails, I promise you that it will happen.

Now let's imagine that instead of sleeping deeply, you simply can't get a good night's sleep—for, say, ten years. At a cellular level, the trillions upon trillions of cells that constitute your body will not receive their much-needed repair. As the years roll by, your nail-producing cells in the matrix will do the best they can under the circumstances, but the best may be dull, soft nails that chip and break. And instead of being rosy, your nails may be pale and grayish from poor circulation. It's possible to think that you have naturally awful nails and that you need some sort of exotic vitamin regimen when what you really need is a good night's sleep. It's also possible to think that your dull, lifeless skin needs an expensive cream or lotion, when sufficient sleep alone would return its radiant glow.

Of course, if you live a busy, deadline-driven life, a good night's sleep may be frustratingly elusive. You have probably already heard many tips for getting a good night's sleep—cutting down on caffeine consumption, buying a good mattress, drinking a cup of warm milk before you go to bed, etc. These are all good suggestions, but I'd like to add some of my own.

Sometimes I think that it's the sheer busyness of modern life that makes getting enough sleep so difficult. It's not realistic to live an insanely busy life and expect to stop on a dime when it's time to sleep. So my advice is to slow down as much as practically possible. Simplify. Stop seeking perfection. Take time to daydream. Occasionally, take time to do nothing at all. Pet a kitten. Stargaze. Throw out all the books that tell you how to do things in fifteen minutes or less. If you can simplify your life and slow it down, gradually, sleep should come more easily. When bedtime arrives, you'll be relaxed and ready to sleep—not feeling that your life is like a team of runaway horses.

Finally, if you continue to be plagued by sleeplessness, don't hesitate to seek professional help. Sleep therapists can help pinpoint any underlying problem, and assist you in establishing good sleep habits.

Getting Sufficient Exercise

Earlier in this chapter, I mentioned how important good circulation is for healthy, beautiful nails. For this reason, exercise is essential. Exercise boosts circulation throughout the entire body, enabling the blood to bring nutrients and oxygen to the nail bed and nail matrix. Without proper circulation, nail beds are pale instead of rosy; nails can be weak and dull; and skin can be dull, dry, and lifeless. Poor circulation can also be the cause of cold hands in the fall and winter months.

Naturally, all exercise is good for your hands and nails. Whatever you can do to get your blood pumping—anything from riding a bicycle to swimming to aerobics—will result in greater hand and nail health. But if you're not now engaged in any regular physical exercise—or even if you are, but you would like to add to your routine—please consider the following circulation-boosting activities.

❑ Take a brisk thirty-minute walk each and every day. This is an easy way to boost circulation. I go for a walk about a half hour after dinner. It's free, it's fun, and you don't have to wear spandex. For at least part of the time, walk as fast as you can.

❑ Stretch like a cat during the day to release the muscle tension that can constrict circulation. Stretching stimulates blood and lymph circulation. In the morning, stretch your entire body from top to bottom before getting out of bed. It feels wonderful! Make up your own stretches, or check your local library for books on stretching. Or observe the nearest cat.

❑ Consider taking a class in yoga. While no one specific yoga posture is especially good for your nails and skin, all yoga postures are beneficial to nail and skin health. The refreshed feeling you have after a yoga practice session is a result of the increased circulation to your brain, as well as the relaxation due to the release of energy from cramped muscles. That same increased blood circulation surges through the capillaries of your fingertips, stimulating nail health and growth. And relaxation of the whole body includes relaxation of the blood vessels in your hands.

❑ Dance. Somewhere along the line, people seem to have forgotten about dancing. It's one of the greatest circulation boosters ever devised. With a partner or without, shut the door, put on some music with a great beat, and dance. You won't want to stop.

❑ To boost upper body circulation, simply rest with your feet and legs above your head for about ten minutes. I do this late in the day when my energy is flagging. You don't need any special equipment for this. Simply lie on the floor and support your feet on your bed or sofa, or rest them on a cushion. You may also want to place cushions under your neck and the small of your back. The blood will flow to the upper part of your body, nourishing your brain and lessening fatigue. For further tension relief, raise your arms above your head and then allow them to fall back behind your head to the floor. You will feel energy flowing to your fingertips.

Following a Proper Diet

Throughout the preceding chapters, I have mentioned the importance of good nutrition to the health of your nails. A number of vitamins, minerals, and other nutrients are needed to build nails that are strong, pliable, and glossy, and to keep skin smooth, healthy, and glowing. When these nutrients are consumed in insufficient amounts, nail and skin health is greatly compromised.

Which nutrients are most important to nail health? All of the B-complex vitamins and vitamins A, C, E, F, and K have been cited by nutritionists as being especially good for nails, with special emphasis on the B vitamin biotin. In Chapter 1, you learned the importance of the mineral sulfur to nails. In fact, sulfur is sometimes called a "beauty mineral" because of its vital role in skin, hair, and nail health. In addition, the minerals iodine, selenium, and zinc are needed in sufficient quantities. Like sulfur, many of these same nutrients are vital for the health of the skin.

Earlier in the book, I mentioned that a specific group of fats is necessary for nail health—and for skin health, as well. This group is called the *essential fatty acids,* or EFAs. These fats are termed essential because, like vitamins and minerals, they must be provided by the diet. Unlike most dietary fat—which can contribute to health problems—the EFAs have been found to be *necessary* for good health. In fact, in the body they work to inhibit the growth of cancer, fight inflammation, and perform many other important functions. Most pertinent to this discussion is that essential fatty acids help keep nails pliable and glossy, and skin smooth and supple.

Are any other nutrients especially important to skin and nail health? Protein contains the amino acids needed to form the cells that build the skin and nails themselves.

At this point, you might be ready to run out and purchase a multivitamin formula that contains all of the vitamins and minerals mentioned above. And, of course, you can also buy supplements of the essential fatty acids and of protein. But fortunately, this isn't necessary. You already have access to the greatest source of nutrition—food! Whole foods—foods that have not been refined or processed—contain a complex array of vitamins, minerals, essential fatty acids, proteins, complex carbohydrates, and much, much more. While a supplement may contain only one nutrient or a handful of nutrients at the most, one food can contain hundreds of beneficial compounds!

So what's the best nutritional advice for someone who's trying to grow the healthiest nails and the most beautiful skin? Eat a balanced diet that includes plenty of whole foods. Fresh fruits and vegetables will provide you with a bounty of vitamins and minerals, as well as a number of other healthful compounds called phytochemicals. Cold-water seafood, flaxseed, and flaxseed oil are the best sources of essential fatty acids. Poultry, meat, eggs, and milk are a few of the foods that contain biotin, sulfur, and the essential amino acids. And remember that your diet should be low in fat, but not fat-free. Some fat is necessary for beautiful hands and nails. (For a more complete list of nail- and skin-healthy foods, see the inset on page 126.)

Sometimes Water Is Good for Your Nails and Skin

In Chapter 1, you learned that by soaking your nails in water while washing dishes or bathing, you can weaken their structure. And experience has probably taught you how frequent exposure to water can harm your skin—especially when the water is combined with drying soaps and detergents. However, healthy nails and skin do naturally contain moisture, and without this moisture, nails become brittle, and skin becomes flaky, dull, and prone to cracking.

To keep your nails pliable and your skin well hydrated, it is important to drink plenty of water throughout the day. Most nutritionists recommend six to eight glasses of water a day. You can verify that you're drinking an adequate amount of water by checking the color of your urine. Dark yellow urine

Eating for Beautiful Hands and Nails

In this chapter, you've learned about the many nutrients that contribute to hand and nail health and beauty. And you've learned that a varied diet which includes plenty of whole foods is the best means of providing your body with the vitamins, minerals, amino acids, and essential fatty acids it needs. But, of course, some foods are higher than others in the specific nutrients required by skin and nails. The following lists will allow you to easily select foods that will provide you with the specific nutrients you want to add to your diet.

Foods Rich in Hand- and Nail-Healthy Vitamins

Apricots
Avocados
Bananas
Beets and beet greens
Blackstrap molasses
Cantaloupe
Chickpeas
Dark green leafy
  vegetables

Mangos
Papayas
Parsley
Peppers
Squash
Sweet potatoes
Wheat germ

Foods Rich in Biotin

Brewer's yeast
Eggs
Liver

Soy products
Whole grains, especially
  barley, millet, and oats

Foods Rich in Sulfur

Apples
Asparagus
Berries
Broccoli
Brussels sprouts
Cabbage
Carrots
Cauliflower
Cherries
Chervil
Cranberries
Cucumbers

Dill
Endive
Figs
Garlic
Gooseberries
Grapes
Horseradish
Leeks
Mustard greens
Onions
Oranges
Parsnips

Foods Rich in Sulfur (continued)

Peaches	Sorrel
Radishes	Spinach
Red cabbage	Watercress
Rutabagas	

Foods Rich in Iodine

Fish, including	Iodized salt
shellfish	Seaweed

Foods Rich in Selenium

Fish, including shellfish	Whole grains
Lean beef, pork, and poultry	

Foods Rich in Zinc

Legumes	shellfish
Seafood, including	Whole grains

Foods Rich in Essential Fatty Acids

Cod	Sardines
Herring	Seeds, especially flax,
Mackerel	pumpkin, and sesame
Nuts, especially hazelnuts	seeds
Salmon	Tuna

Foods Rich in Protein

Beans	Lean beef, pork, and poultry
Fish, including	Low-fat dairy products
shellfish	Tofu

indicates that you should drink more water. Clear urine that looks almost like water indicates that you may be overdoing it. Of course, your weight and physical activity, as well as the season of the year, can all affect the amount of water you need on a daily basis.

There is really so much you can do to make your hands and nails stronger and more attractive. Proper nail care, adequate exercise, sufficient rest, a good diet—all can help you have healthier, lovelier nails and smoother, more radiant skin. As a bonus, many of these practices contribute to general health, leading to greater energy and an all-over glow. What could be more beautiful?

Conclusion

Do You Have Time for Beautiful Hands and Nails?

I don't know about you, but there are times when I feel that too many people in the media are telling me that if I devote just five minutes a day to this or ten minutes a day to that, I can be so much better—thinner, more beautiful, whatever—than I am now. Just five minutes a day to rock-hard abs! Just three minutes to banishing cellulite! And on and on. By now, you may be thinking, "But I have no time to do even what I'm doing *now*. How am I going to work a hand- and nail-care regimen into my life?"

This is certainly a good question, and it deserves a good answer. Let me start by saying that I perform the Beautiful Hands and Nails Regimen every day, cleaning, protecting, and nourishing my nails on an ongoing basis. It's quick, it's easy, and it's the first line of defense against damage caused by time, weather, and everyday activities. I find that I can easily incorporate the regimen into my morning routine—which is not to say that on every morning, I spend the same amount of time on my nails. On busy days, the bare bones regimen is all I have time for. But if that day includes some type of special event, I buff my nails, using two thin layers of buffing cream, and *then* apply the nail protector. This lends my nails a soft, translucent sheen. Then I massage in my hand cream—one containing sunscreen, of course—and I'm ready to go!

During the day, I use my hand- and nail-care products as needed, or whenever I have the time. If I'm doing housework, I may use the nail protector twice a day or more. I also usually rub beeswax onto the filed edges of my nails to protect them from the caustic effects of cleansers. And if a nail begins to chip or split as I do my chores, I quickly apply my Beeswax Nail Spackle, which is a real lifesaver for fragile nails like mine.

I keep a small jar of medicated petroleum jelly on the windowsill above the kitchen sink, and rub it in every time I wash dishes. Or, if I have lots of dishes to do, I wear rubber gloves. This underscores an important rule of nail care: Have your nail-care supplies dotted about the house, at work, and in your car—*everywhere* you might need them. If you have to go hunting for your nail-care supplies, nail care becomes a chore, and is often bypassed in the rush of the day.

By the seat in our TV room, I keep a small basket containing nail files, a hindostone, a cuticle trimmer, a cube of beeswax, buffing cream and buffer, and other miscellaneous nail paraphernalia. Then, while watching television, I devote a few minutes to my nails. Even if you watch very little television, you will have enough time to maintain nail shape, file off any rough edges, and repair any damage done since your morning routine.

Finally, before going to bed, I use my nail nourisher, varying what I use depending on my mood and what my nails seem to need. This takes only a minute or two.

I use more intensive hand treatments every week and a half to two weeks, but I am not rigid about this. In the dead of winter, though, I do use the Intensive Moisturizing Treatment once or twice weekly. Without it, my hands would suffer. I also may use the Bran Hand Softener or the Warm Paraffin Hand Treatment, partly to get my hands warm on a cold day. This highlights a nice thing about hand treatments—they *feel* so good! And you can feel good about using all of the treatments in this book because they're nondrying and nontoxic. No formaldehyde. No toluene. No methyl methacrylate. Just wholesome, natural substances that will nourish and protect your nails and hands with a minimum of fuss, bother, and expense.

Are the results worth the time and effort? To this, I answer with an emphatic *yes*! I have already described how much these treatments have improved the condition of my own hands and nails. Never again will I feel embarrassed by reddened skin, roughened calluses, or dry, chipped nails. I get a special kick out of having attractive hands after so many years of having horrible ones! I think you, too, will find these treatments easy, effective, and fun. I wish you the best.

Resource List

Many of the natural products used in the treatments and therapies in this book are readily available at local drugstores, health foods stores, and hobby stores. If you are unable to locate any of the ingredients needed, however, the following list can guide you to a manufacturer who can sell the product to you directly.

Avalon Skin Care Products, Inc.
499 Wright Street, #301
Lakewood, CO 80228-1105
(888) 295–OILS
Essential oils.

Lavender Lane
7337 #1 Roseville Road
Sacramento, CA 95842
(916) 334–4400
Alkanet powder; beeswax; essential oils; lanolin; sweet almond oil; jojoba oil; and jars and bottles.

Moonrise Herbs
826 G Street
Arcata, CA 95521

(800) 603–8364
Alkanet powder; calendula flowers; and henna.

Penn Herb Co. Ltd.
10601 Decatur Road, Suite #2
Philadelphia, PA 19154-3293
(800) 523–9971
Alkanet powder; beeswax; dried calendula flowers; myrrh oil; orris root powder; and henna.

Soap Saloon
5710 Auburn Boulevard #6
Sacramento, CA 95841
(916) 334–4894
Beeswax.

Bibliography

Balch, James F., MD, and Phyllis A. Balch, CNC. *Prescription for Nutritional Healing: A Practical A–Z Reference to Drug-Free Remedies Using Vitamins, Minerals, Herbs & Food Supplements.* Garden City Park, NY: Avery Publishing Group, 1997.

Braverman, Eric R., MD, with Carl C. Pfeiffer, MD. *The Healing Nutrients Within: Facts, Findings and New Research on Amino Acids.* New Canaan, CT: Keats Publishing, 1987.

Crayhon, Robert, MS. *Robert Crayhon's Nutrition Made Simple.* New York: Evans and Company, 1994.

Deutsch, Ronald M., and Judi S. Morrill. *Realities of Nutrition.* Palo Alto, CA: Bull Publishing, 1993.

Diamond, Marilyn. *The American Vegetarian Cookbook From the Fit for Life Kitchen.* New York: Warner Books, 1990.

Gallery, David, ND. "Surphur: Nature's 'Beauty Mineral.'" *Let's Live* (June 1990).

Gerras, Charles, Editor. *Feasting on Raw Foods.* Emmaus, PA: Rodale Press, 1980.

Gorton, Annie. "The New Age of Natural Manicures." *Nails* (June 1992).

Haas, Elson M., MD. *Staying Healthy With Nutrition.* New York: Evans and Company, 1994.

Jensen, Bernard. *Foods That Heal.* Garden City Park, NY: Avery Publishing Group, 1988.

Jensen, Bernard. *Vital Foods for Total Health.* Solana Beach, CA: Bernard Jensen Products, 1984.

Keller, Erich. *Aromatherapy Handbook for Beauty, Hair, and Skin Care.* Rochester, VT: Healing Arts Press, 1991.

Kushi, Aveline, Wendy Esko, and Maya Tiwari. *Diet for Natural Beauty: A Natural Anti-Aging Formula for Skin & Hair Care.* Tokyo and New York: Japan Publications, 1991.

Miller, E.P. "The Modern Manicure." *Self* (April 1993).

Napier, John. *Hands.* New York: Pantheon Books, 1980.

Nordberg, Marie. "Habitual Rituals." *Nailpro* (June 1992).

Rudin, Donald O., MD, and Clara Felix. *Omega 3 Oils: To Improve Mental Health, Fight Degenerative Diseases, and Extend Your Life.* Garden City Park, NY: Avery Publishing Group, 1996.

Samman, Peter D., and David A. Fenton. *The Nails in Disease.* 4th ed. Chicago: William Heinemann Medical Books, 1986.

Stitt, Paul A. *Why George Should Eat Broccoli.* Milwaukee: The Dougherty Company, 1990.

Tabori, Paul. *The Book of the Hand.* Philadelphia, PA: Chilton, 1962.

Tisserand, Robert B. *The Art of Aromatherapy.* Rochester, VT: Healing Arts Press, 1977.

Traven, Beatrice. *The Complete Book of Natural Cosmetics.* Paramus, NJ: Simon and Schuster, 1974.

Wilson, Roberta. *Aromatherapy for Vibrant Health and Beauty: A Practical A to Z Reference to Aromatherapy Treatments for Health, Skin, and Hair Problems Using Essential Oils.* Garden City Park, NY: Avery Publishing Group, 1995.

Index

Grapefruit Oil Soother,
   Fresh, 55
Grip
   power, 18
   precision, 18

H

Hand and Arm De-Ager, 112
Hand and nail problems,
   troubleshooting for, 9–16
Hand Butter, 37
Hand care, 91–112
   and exercise, 94
   intensive, 102–104
   preventive, 92–95
   regimen. *See* Beautiful
   Hands and Nails
   Regimen.
   rehabilitative, 98–112
Hand softeners, 98–105
   Bran Hand Softener, 98–99
   Cornmeal and Olive Oil
      Exfoliating Treatment, 100
   Egg White Hand Mask, 99
   Intensive Moisturizing
      Treatment, 101
   Lavender Hand Wash, 99
   Oatmeal Softening
      Treatment, 100
   Simple Papaya Hand
      Treatment, 100–101
   Warm Paraffin Hand
      Treatment, 104–105
   White Glove Treatment,
      The, 101–104

Hands, anatomy of, 18–19
Hands and Nails Regimen,
   Beautiful, 29–45
Hangnails, 12, 23
   treating, 32–33, 42, 58–59
Henna
   to color nails, 84–87
   to harden nails, 85
Hindostone, 50, 63
Honey and Lemon Smoother,
   109

I

Intensive Moisturizing
   Treatment, 101
Iodine
   foods rich in, 127
   importance of, 124

J

Jojoba oil, 31

K

Keratin, 23, 24–25

L

Lanolin, 32, 33–34
Lavender Cuticle Soother,
   54–55

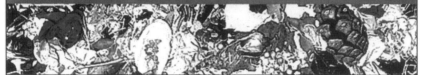

A PRACTICAL A TO Z REFERENCE TO AROMATHERAPY TREATMENTS
FOR HEALTH, SKIN, AND HAIR PROBLEMS USING ESSENTIAL OILS

A COMPLETE GUIDE TO UNDERSTANDING & USING

AROMATHERAPY

FOR VIBRANT HEALTH & BEAUTY

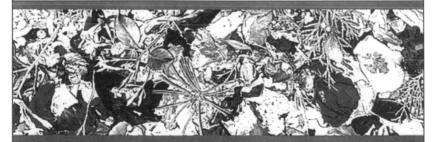

ROBERTA WILSON

0-89529-627-6 • $13.95

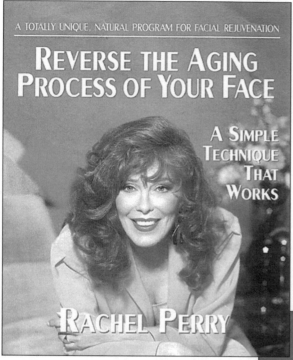

A TOTALLY UNIQUE, NATURAL PROGRAM FOR FACIAL REJUVENATION

REVERSE THE AGING PROCESS OF YOUR FACE

A SIMPLE TECHNIQUE THAT WORKS

RACHEL PERRY

0-89529-625-X • $13.95

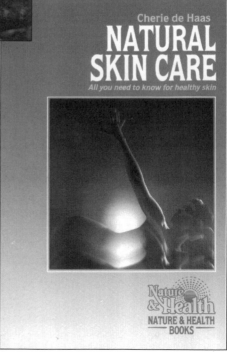

Cherie de Haas

NATURAL SKIN CARE

All you need to know for healthy skin

NATURE & HEALTH BOOKS

0-89529-400-1 • $8.95

Healthy Habits
are easy to come by—
If You Know Where to Look!

To get the latest information on:
- better health • diet & weight loss
- the latest nutritional supplements
- herbal healing & homeopathy and more

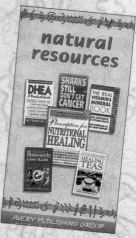

COMPLETE AND RETURN THIS CARD RIGHT AWAY!

Where did you purchase this book?

❏ bookstore   ❏ health food store   ❏ pharmacy
❏ supermarket   ❏ other (please specify)_____

Name _____

Street Address _____

City _____ State _____ Zip _____

Trying to eat healthier? Looking to lose weight? Frustrated with bland-tasting fat-free foods?

For more information on how you can create low-fat
meals that are packed with taste and nutrition and develop
healthy habits that can improve the quality of your life,

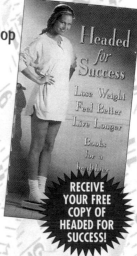

COMPLETE AND RETURN THIS CARD!

Where did you purchase this book?

❏ bookstore   ❏ health food store   ❏ pharmacy
❏ supermarket   ❏ other (please specify)_____

Name _____

Street Address _____

City _____ State _____ Zip _____

RECEIVE
YOUR FREE
COPY OF
HEADED FOR
SUCCESS!

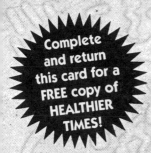

PLACE
STAMP
HERE

AVERY PUBLISHING GROUP
120 Old Broadway
Garden City Park, NY 11040

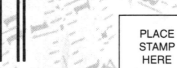

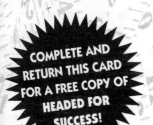
PLACE
STAMP
HERE

AVERY PUBLISHING GROUP
120 Old Broadway
Garden City Park, NY 11040